Novel Insights on Oral Anticoagulants in Clinical Practice Focus on Acenocoumarol

Novel Insights on Oral Anticoagulants in Clinical Practice

Focus on Acenocoumarol

Editor

Jagdish Hiremath DM DNB
Interventional Cardiologist
Director, Cath Lab
Department of Cardiology
Ruby Hall Clinic
Pune, Maharashtra, India

Foreword

Jamshed Dalal

JAYPEE
The Health Sciences Publisher
New Delhi | London | Panama

Jaypee Brothers Medical Publishers (P) Ltd

Headquarters

Jaypee Brothers Medical Publishers (P) Ltd
4838/24, Ansari Road, Daryaganj
New Delhi 110 002, India
Phone: +91-11-43574357
Fax: +91-11-43574314
Email: jaypee@jaypeebrothers.com

Overseas Offices

J.P. Medical Ltd
83 Victoria Street, London
SW1H 0HW (UK)
Phone: +44 20 3170 8910
Fax: +44 (0)20 3008 6180
Email: info@jpmedpub.com

Jaypee-Highlights Medical Publishers Inc
City of Knowledge, Bld. 237, Clayton
Panama City, Panama
Phone: +1 507-301-0496
Fax: +1 507-301-0499
Email: cservice@jphmedical.com

Jaypee Brothers Medical Publishers (P) Ltd
17/1-B Babar Road, Block-B, Shaymali
Mohammadpur, Dhaka-1207
Bangladesh
Mobile: +08801912003485
Email: jaypeedhaka@gmail.com

Jaypee Brothers Medical Publishers (P) Ltd
Bhotahity, Kathmandu
Nepal
Phone: +977-9741283608
Email: kathmandu@jaypeebrothers.com

Website: www.jaypeebrothers.com
Website: www.jaypeedigital.com

Novel Insights on Oral Anticoagulants
in Clinical Practice: Focus on Acenocoumarol / Jagdish Hiremath

First Edition: **2018**

ISBN: 978-93-5270-023-3

Printed at: Paras Offset Pvt. Ltd., New Delhi

KEY POINTS

- The association between patient education and superior anticoagulation control is well established
- Educating patients on factors affecting their time in therapeutic range and methods to manage their anticoagulant therapy may result in increased compliance to the therapeutic regimen
- Continuous counseling and increasing patient awareness of various aspects of anticoagulant therapy will result in improved therapeutic outcomes
- Technological advances in the form of point-of-care devices have improved self-management of anticoagulant therapy
- Self-testing and self-monitoring (using at-home international normalized ratio monitoring devices such as the CoaguChek® monitor), besides being convenient, have several advantages, including better patient adherence, more frequent monitoring, and fewer complications.

REFERENCES

1. Trailokya A. Role of patient education and counseling in acenocoumarol management. Intern Med. 2016;6:2012.
2. Clarkesmith DE, Pattison HM, Lane DA. Educational and behavioural interventions for anticoagulant therapy in patients with atrial fibrillation. Cochrane Database Syst Rev. 2013;6:CD008600.
3. Tang EO, Lai CS, Lee KK, Wong RS, Cheng G, Chan TY. Relationship between patients' warfarin knowledge and anticoagulation control. Ann Pharmacother. 2003;37:34-9.
4. Ibrahim R, Saber-Ayad M. Continuous outpatient warfarin counseling and its effects on adherence. Asian J Pharm Clin Res. 2013;6:101-4.
5. Garcia-Alamino JM, Ward AM, Alonso-Coello P, Perera R, Bankhead C, Fitzmaurice D, et al. Self-monitoring and self-management of oral anticoagulation. Cochrane Database Syst Rev. 2010;(4):CD003839.
6. Heneghan C, Alonso-Coello P, Garcia-Alamino JM, Perera R, Glasziou P. Self-monitoring of oral anticoagulation: a systematic review and meta-analysis. Lancet. 2006;367:404-11.
7. Meneghelo ZM, Barroso CM, Liporace IL, Cora AP. Comparison of the international normalized ratio levels obtained by portable coagulometer and laboratory in a clinic specializing in oral anticoagulation. Int J Lab Hematol. 2015;37:536-43.
8. Gardiner C, Williams K, Mackie IJ, Machin SJ, Cohen H. Patient self-testing is a reliable and acceptable alternative to laboratory INR monitoring. Br J Haematol. 2005;128:242-7.
9. Havrda DE, Hawk TL, Marvin CM. Accuracy and precision of the CoaguChek S versus laboratory INRs in a clinic. Ann Pharmacother. 2002;36:769-75.
10. Shiach CR, Campbell B, Poller L, Keown M, Chauhan N. Reliability of point-of-care prothrombin time testing in a community clinic: a randomized crossover comparison with hospital laboratory testing. Br J Haematol. 2002;119(2):370-75.
11. Legacyhealth. Vitamin K and warfarin guidelines. [online] Available from: https://www.legacyhealth.org/. [Accessed February, 2017].

Contributors

Editor

Jagdish Hiremath DM DNB
Interventional Cardiologist
Director, Cath Lab
Department of Cardiology
Ruby Hall Clinic
Pune, Maharashtra, India

Contributing Authors

Rajiv Agarwal MD DM
Interventional Cardiologist
Department of Cardiology
New Delhi, India

Yugandhar Bachhu MD DM FACC FESC
Interventional Cardiologist
Department of Cardiology
Sri Venkata Sai Hrudayalaya
Tirupati, Andhra Pradesh, India

Deependra Bhatnagar DM DNB MD FSCAI FESC
Interventional Cardiologist
Additional Director-Cardiology
Department of Cardiology
Fortis Escorts Hospital
Jaipur, Rajasthan, India

Mrinal K Das MD DM FICC FCSI
Consultant and Interventional Cardiologist
Department of Cardiology
BM Birla Heart Research Centre
Kolkata, West Bengal, India

Sanjay Dhaded MS MCH
Senior Consultant Cardiac Surgeon
Department of CVTS
Narayana Institute of Cardiac Sciences
Bangalore, Karnataka, India

SK Goel MD FACC FESC DM
Cardiologist
Department of Cardiology
Shantideep Hospital
Bulandshahr, Uttar Pradesh, India

Uday M Jadhav MD FACC FESC FCAPSC FICC FIAE FISE FCSI FICP
Consultant
Department of Cardiology
MGM New Bombay Hospital
Mumbai, Maharashtra, India

Nazir I Juvale MD DM MNAMS FACC FSCAI FESC
Consultant
Department of Cardiology
Saifee Hospital
Mumbai, Maharashtra, India

Ummer K MD DM
Interventional Neurologist
Department of Neurology
Baby Memorial Hospital
Calicut, Kerala, India

Sridhar Kasturi MD DM FACC FSCAI
Senior Consultant Interventional Cardiologist
Department of Cardiology
Sunshine Heart Institute
Secunderabad, Telangana, India

B Kesavamoorthy MD DM
Senior Consultant Cardiology
Cardiology Clinic
Tanjore, Tamil Nadu, India

K Damodara Rao Kodem MD DM
Consultant Interventional Cardiologist
Department of Cardiology
My Cure Hospitals
Visakhapatnam, Andhra Pradesh, India

Nirmal Kumar MD DM FSCAI FESC
Consultant Cardiologist
Department of Cardiology
Care Hospitals
Hyderabad, Telangana, India

Nitin S Patki MD DM FACC FESC
Interventional Cardiologist
Department of Cardiology
NM Wadia Institute of Cardiology
Pune, Maharashtra, India

Prasant K Sahoo MD DM FRCP FACC FSCAI FESC FAPSIC FICC FCSI FISE FIAE
Senior Consultant Cardiologist
Director Interventional Cardiology
Department of Cardiology
Apollo Hospitals
Bhubaneswar, Orissa, India

Bhupesh Shah MD DM
Associate Professor and Interventional Cardiologist
Department of Cardiology, VS Hospital
Ahmedabad, Gujarat, India

Yogendra Singh MD DM FSCAI
Consultant Interventional Cardiology
Department of Cardiology
Fortis Escorts Hospital
Dehradun, Uttarakhand, India

Prashant Vaijyanath MS MCH FACS FCS
Director
Department of Cardiothoracic Surgery
Kovai Medical Center and Hospital
Limited, Coimbatore, Tamil Nadu, India

Foreword

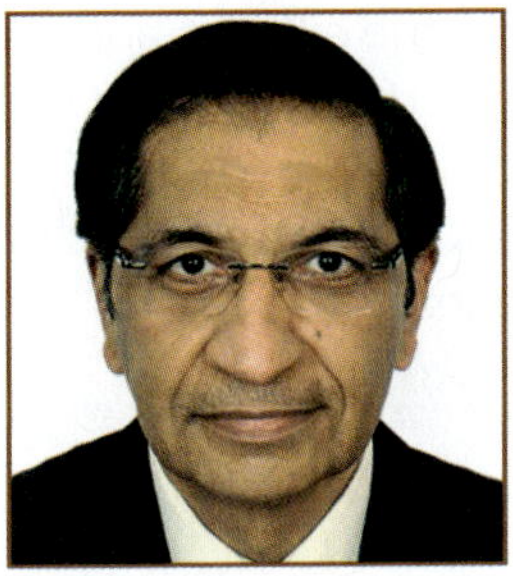

Jamshed Dalal MBBS MD DM PhD FESC FRCP
Director, Cardiac Sciences
Kokilaben Dhirubhai Ambani Hospital
Mumbai, Maharashtra, India

We all know how a rat poison, warfarin, became a life-saving drug and are surprised that even today it continues to be so widely used after its discovery nearly 60 years ago. The importance of anticoagulation in medicine, in 1953, led to the development of another oral anticoagulant, acenocoumarol, which has several advantages over warfarin and has been extensively discussed in this book. These two drugs remained the mainstay in maintaining anticoagulation in a variety of situations such as artificial valves, atrial fibrillation, deep vein thrombosis, pulmonary embolism, and any condition that requires blood thinning. Warfarin and acenocoumarol remain remarkably cheap drugs but do have the disadvantage of needing close monitoring and dose adjustments due to interaction with some foods and other drugs. After more than half a century, a new variety of anticoagulants, called novel or nonvitamin K oral anticoagulants (NOACs) have been developed. However, in certain specific conditions, such as metallic prosthetic valves, the earlier anticoagulants still have to be used.

Bringing out this book, which is an extensive and exhausting review on anticoagulation and vitamin K antagonists, takes foresight. I give credit to all those involved in understanding the continued importance of these original molecules in the face of development of NOACs. Due to issues of cost and other important factors, the original anticoagulants still remain today the most frequently used oral anticoagulants in the world and are likely to remain so for a considerable time in the future. Any doctor whoever needs to prescribe an oral anticoagulant must read this book to get a full understanding of the whole subject of anticoagulation and its treatment.

Dr Jagdish Hiremath, who has edited this book, is the perfect person to do so, having extensive experience in all fields of clinical and intervention cardiology. I personally know Dr Hiremath for several decades from a budding cardiologist to an internationally renowned interventional cardiologist. I am fortunate enough to meet him at several conferences across the world as he travels from Pune to head several meetings, advisory boards, and teaching sessions. He has drawn upon a galaxy of national stalwarts to write the different chapters and each one has done an exemplary job of bringing out the nuances of each topic from and overview of coagulation and hemostasis to details of these drugs in a variety of clinical situations.

I am sure this book will remain an important work on the subject and be a boon for both students appearing for exams to the expert looking for finer points. I compliment every one involved in initiating this project and making available to the medical community a comprehensive book providing extensive knowledge on the whole process of anticoagulation and its management.

Preface

Anticoagulation has been a major cardiological therapy for more than 60 years. In variety of clinical situations, anticoagulations have formed the backbone of treatment. Over a period of nearly 60 years, the evolution has been quite slow. The original coumadin derivatives continue to rule the roost in valvular heart disease, structural heart disease with atrial fibrillation, deep vein thrombosis and other thrombotic diseases.

If used judiciously and in awareness, the coumadin derivatives can effectively treat these thrombotic conditions. The awareness related to anticoagulations, their complications, and investigations have evolved over time. However, effective implementation has remained as weak as in the past. With newer laboratories, more precise prothrombin time reports, and easy communications, we should be able to offer our patients highly scientific anticoagulation.

This book rolls out all the intricacies related to anticoagulation. The nitty-gritty of pharmacological actions, investigations, dose adjustments, and complications are all put under one cover. This will be a ready reference book for all the practitioners who use anticoagulants. The role of newer anticoagulants has been emerging for the last 5 years. In India, the growth is limited by the cost factor. Coumadin derivatives continue to be cost-effective.

This book will further enhance the knowledge base of practitioners and help us effectively offer this tricky, yet highly cost-effective treatment to our patients.

Jagdish Hiremath

Acknowledgments

I would like to begin with a heartfelt thank you to all the authors of the book. Each of them, being an expert in their field, have contributed enormously to the making of this book. Indeed, it is their tireless dedication to this project in spite of their busy schedule that has ensured that this textbook has come out so well.

I would also like to thank Dr Vikrama Raja for being the collaborator and efficiently supporting me in this project.

A special thanks to the team at M/s Jaypee Brothers Medical Publishers (P) Ltd., for their technical expertise and bringing out this book in such creative and aesthetically appealing manner.

Contents

1

Overview of Coagulation and Hemostasis

Jagdish Hiremath, Prasant K Sahoo

INTRODUCTION

This chapter provides information on the coagulation cascade, and intrinsic and extrinsic coagulation pathways. The chapter also highlights the three phases of coagulation as well as regulatory mechanisms involved in the coagulatory process.

OVERVIEW OF HEMOSTASIS

Hemostasis is a highly conserved mechanism that allows the human body to repair damaged blood vessels, maintain the fluid state of blood, and remove blood clots after the restoration of vascular integrity (Fig. 1). Coagulation, commonly known as blood clotting, plays an essential role in hemostasis.[1]

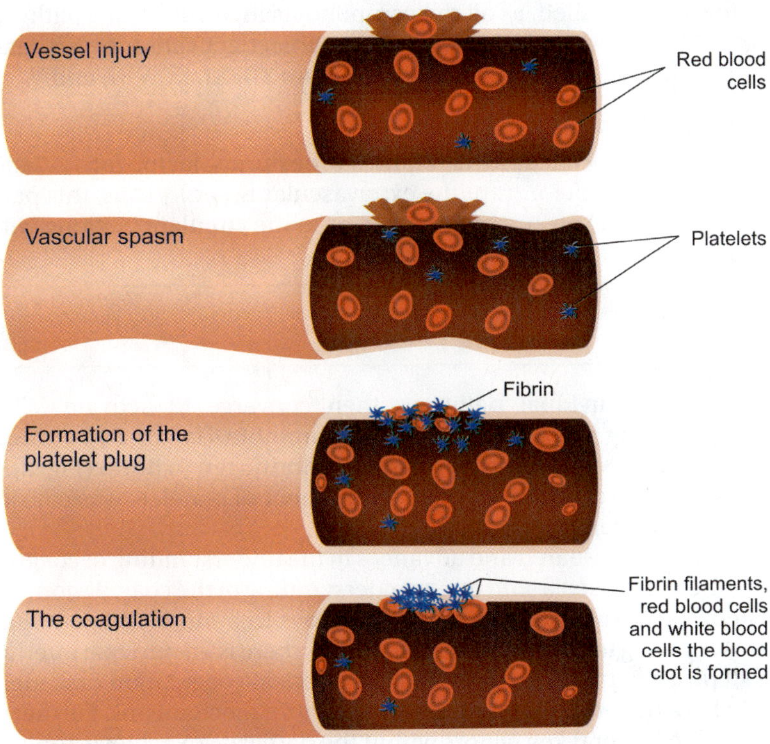

Fig. 1: The process of hemostasis.[1]

Coagulation plays an essential role in hemostasis.[1]

Coagulation Cascade

The coagulation cascade was proposed in 1964 as a series of coordinated enzymatic conversions. The coagulation cascade was explained as a stepwise interaction of clotting factors with one another, resulting in activation of these factors and consequently, the formation of fibrin.[2] The important coagulation proteins are listed in table 1.[3]

Table 1: Proteins involved in the coagulation process[3]

Fibinogen	Vitamin K-dependent	Contact
Fibrinogen	Factor II	Factor XII
Factor V	Factor VII	HMWK*
Factor VIII	Factor IX	Prekallikrein**
Factor XIII	Factor X	Factor XI

*HMWK, hight-molecular weight kininogen, also known as fitzgerald factor.
**known as Fletcher factor.

The coagulation cascade has been described under two pathways, viz., the (i) intrinsic and (ii) extrinsic pathways.[2]

Intrinsic Pathway

This pathway is so called, as all the components involved in this pathway are present in the blood.[1] It is dependent on contact activation by a negatively charged surface. It involves coagulation factors XII, XI, IX, VIII, and V.[2]

Extrinsic Pathway

This pathway is so called, as it requires an external factor for initiation of coagulation (tissue factor from the extravascular tissue).[1] Thus, this pathway is triggered by the exposure of tissue factor to the circulation; along with the tissue factor, this pathway involves factor VII.[2]

The coagulation cascade is widely described by two pathways, viz., the intrinsic and extrinsic pathways.

Both these individual pathways then converge to activate factor X, ultimately causing the conversion of prothrombin (factor II) to thrombin (factor IIa). This results in the conversion of fibrinogen to fibrin (Fig. 2).[2]

In this cascade model, the initial recruitment of platelets was considered to be an independent mechanism.[2]

With the latest research and advances in the understanding of coagulation process, there has been a shift in the understanding of the coagulation process from stepwise intrinsic and extrinsic pathways to a more all-encompassing model. According to the latest understanding, there is an intricate interlinking of the stepwise patterns explained in the classical coagulation cascade. Now there is also a better understanding of regulatory mechanisms. Furthermore, the potency of several key factors within the pathway, to achieve appropriate and regulated hemostasis, is also better understood.[2]

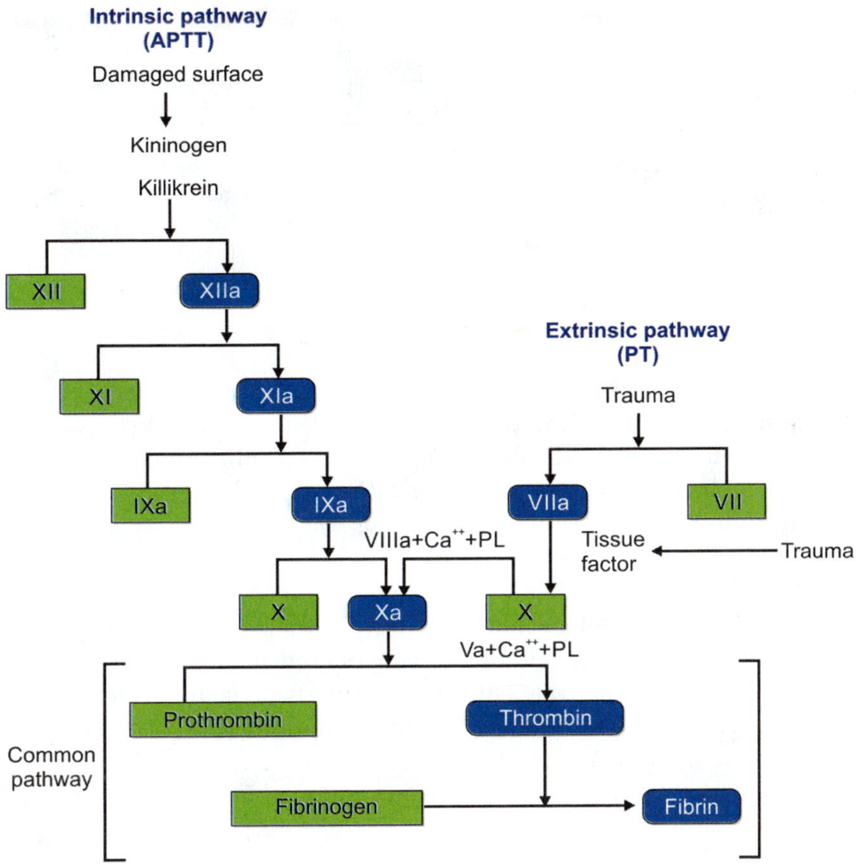

Fig. 2: Classic coagulation cascade[2]

Source: Adams RL, Bird RJ. Review article: Coagulation cascade and therapeutics update: relevance to nephrology. Part 1: Overview of coagulation, thrombophilias and history of anticoagulants. Nephrology (Carlton). 2009; 14(5):462-70.

> Three phases of coagulation include:
> 1. Initiation phase, 2. Amplification phase, 3. Propagation phase

Three Phases of Coagulation

While the coagulation cascade has been commonly used to understand the process of coagulation, a cell biological model of coagulation is also gaining attention. According to this current model of coagulation, the process can be divided into three separate phases (Fig. 3).[1]

Initiation Phase

Classically known as the extrinsic phase, the initiation phase begins with the exposure of subendothelial cells and fibroblasts to the blood stream due to the damage to the vasculature. With this, a key initiator of the coagulation cascade, tissue factor, is exposed. Tissue factor acts

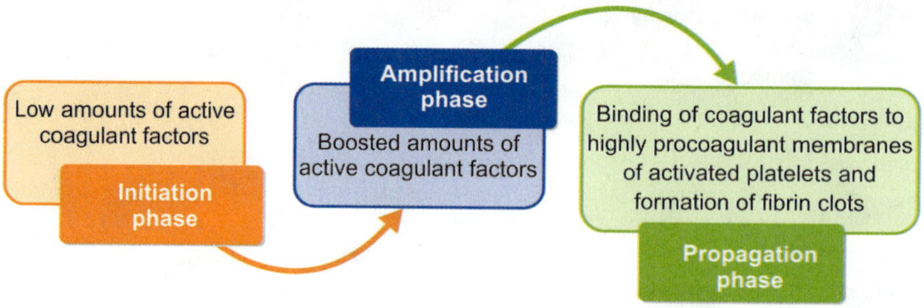

Fig. 3: Phases of coagulation[1]

as a cofactor for factor VII and activates it to VIIa. The tissue factor/VIIa complex also produces traces of factors IXa and Xa. Factor Xa then associates with the cofactor, factor Va, to form a prothrombinase complex on tissue factor—expressing cells; this ultimately leads to the conversion of prothrombin (factor II) to thrombin (Fig. 4).[1]

Amplification Phase

The thrombin produced in the initiation phase, though low in quantity, keeps activating the platelets that have gathered in the region of injury. Parallelly, thrombin activates the platelet-derived factor V to Va. This further amplifies prothrombinase activity, and also activates factor VIII to VIIIa. Activated factor VIIIa acts as a cofactor to factor IXa on the surface of activated platelets and supports the activation of factor X. Furthermore, thrombin also activates factor XI to XIa.[1]

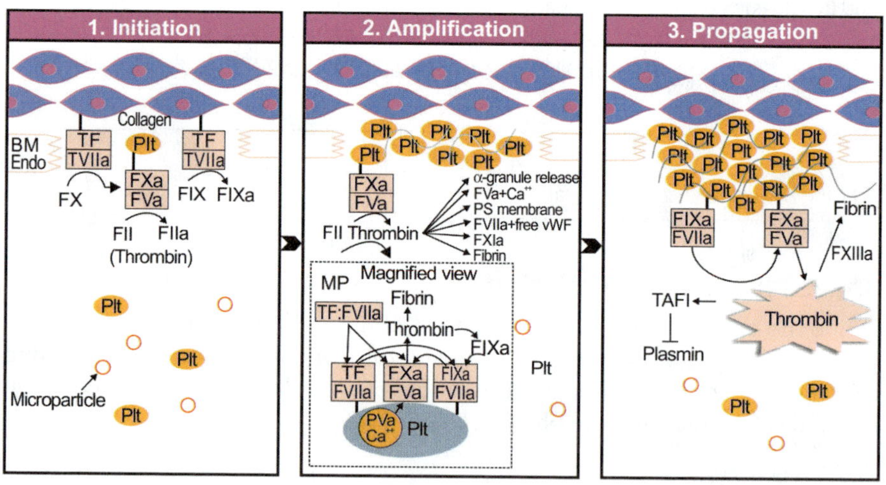

TF, tissue factor; FVIIa, recombinant factor VII; Plt, Platelet; FXa, factor Xa; FVa, factor Va; FVIIa, factor VIIa; FIX, factor IXa; TAFI, thrombin-activatable fibrinolysis inhibitor; PS, prothrombinase.

Fig. 4: Mechanisms involved in different phases of coagulation[2]

Propagation Phase

The propagation phase takes place on surfaces of activated platelets, which contain procoagulant phospholipids. Activated factor XIa further activates factor IX to IXa, which then associates with thrombin-cleaved factor VIII. On phosphatidylserine-exposing cell membranes, the tenase complex of activated factors IXa/VIIIa helps in the activation of factor X to Xa. The factor Xa/Va complex then produces adequate quantities of thrombin to form fibrin fibers. Finally, the thrombin-activated factor XIIIa helps in the formation of covalent crosslinks between fibrin chains to form an elastic, polymerized fibrin clot.[1]

Fibrinolysis

The removal of the clot by fibrinolysis is essential, both following the formation of a clot in response to vascular damage or due to pathological thrombosis (arterial or venous), and atherosclerosis. Fibrinolysis is primarily mediated by plasmin, which is produced by the proteolytic cleavage of circulating plasminogen by two main effectors:[2]

1. Tissue-type plasminogen activator (released from endothelial cells in response to thrombin and venous occlusion)
2. Urokinase-type plasminogen activator [secreted as prourokinase, and activated by plasmin and contact factors (kininogen, prekallikrein, and factor XII)]

Inappropriate plasmin generation is prevented by the abundance of plasminogen activator inhibitors in the flowing blood. These plasminogen activator inhibitors form inactivating complexes with the tissue-type and urokinase-type plasminogen activators explained above.[2]

Plasmin cleaves fibrin at specific lysine and arginine residues, resulting in the production of fibrin degradation products.[2]

Each level and phase of the coagulation process is regulated by inhibitory factors.

REGULATION OF COAGULATION

Each level and phase of the coagulation process is regulated by inhibitory factors, either by enzymatic inhibition or by modulation of cofactor activity. Various regulatory proteins of the coagulation cascade and their point of action are summarized in table 2.[2]

Table 2: Regulatory proteins of the coagulation cascade[2]

Regulatory protein	Expression	Substrate
Tissue factor pathway inhibitor	• Endothelium • Platelets • LDL bound (circulating)	• TF-factor VIIa • Factor Xa

Continued

Continued

Table 2: Regulatory proteins of the coagulation cascade[2]

Regulatory protein	Expression	Substrate
Antithrombin	• Endothelium	• Free serine proteases • Bound serine proteases (less)
Heparin cofactor II (+ heparin)	• Liver	• Thrombin
Thrombomodulin	• Endothelium	• Factor V/Va • Factor VIII/VIIIa
Protein C + cofactor protein S	• Liver	• Factor V/Va • Factor VIII/VIIIa
Protein Z-dependent protease inhibitor	• Liver	• Factor Xa
α1-protease inhibitor	• Liver	• Factor Xa thrombin
α2-macroglobulin	• Liver	• Thrombin factor Xa • Plasmin • Kallikreins

LDL, low-density lipoprotein.

KEY POINTS

- Coagulation is an integral part of hemostasis
- The process of coagulation has been classically explained as a coagulation cascade, wherein a stepwise activation of clotting factors leads to the formation of a fibrin clot
- The current cell biological model of coagulation explains the process in three phases, viz. (i) initiation, (ii) amplification, and (iii) propagation
- Once the vasculature has been repaired, fibrinolysis is mediated by plasmin
- The coagulation process is regulated at each step and level by various inhibitory factors.

REFERENCES

1. Versteeg HH, Heemskerk JW, Levi M, Reitsma PH. New fundamentals in hemostasis. Physiol Rev. 2013;93(1):327-58.
2. Adams RL, Bird RJ. Review article: Coagulation cascade and therapeutics update: relevance to nephrology. Part 1: Overview of coagulation, thrombophilias and history of anticoagulants. Nephrology (Carlton). 2009;14(5):462-70.
3. Triplett DA. Coagulation and bleeding disorders: review and update. Clin Chem. 2000;46(8 Pt 2):1260-9.

2

Anticoagulants: Oral and Parenteral Agents

SK Goel

INTRODUCTION

Heparins and coumarins have been the mainstay of anticoagulant therapy for over 60 years. The anticoagulant properties of heparin were first discovered by McLean in 1915 during his search for a procoagulant in the dog liver, and in 1930 Link identified dicoumarol as the causative agent of sweet clover disease, a hemorrhagic condition in cattle.[1] Several medical conditions require management through anticoagulation therapy. Anticoagulation therapy is indicated in patients with venous thromboembolism (VTE) and ischemic stroke, for the prevention of recurrent thrombosis.[2] In addition, conditions such as atrial fibrillation, cardioversion, vascular heart disease, myocardial infarction, and anti-phospholipid syndrome may also require anticoagulation.[3]

In this chapter, we will discuss anticoagulants used in clinical practice, their classification, sites of action in the coagulation cascade, and anticoagulants in the developmental pipeline. This chapter provides information on the classification of anticoagulants and sites of action of these agents within the coagulation cascade. This chapter also highlights novel oral and parenteral anticoagulants in the pipeline.

CLASSIFICATION OF ANTICOAGULANTS

Based on the route of administration, anticoagulants can be classified as oral and parenteral. Further, anticoagulants can also be classified according to the site of action in the coagulation cascade (Fig. 1).[4] Conventional anticoagulant therapies include parenteral heparins and oral vitamin K antagonists (VKAs), such as acenocoumarol and warfarin.[5]

> Anticoagulants can be broadly classified as oral and parenteral, based on the route of administration.

Anticoagulants such as low molecular weight heparins (LMWHs) (e.g., enoxaparin), and fondaparinux have relatively discrete targets in the coagulation pathway. Despite having potential benefits over VKAs, they require parenteral administration and are substantially more expensive than VKAs. Further, newer anticoagulants, such as dabigatran, rivaroxaban, and apixaban, have specific targets (Fig. 2).[5]

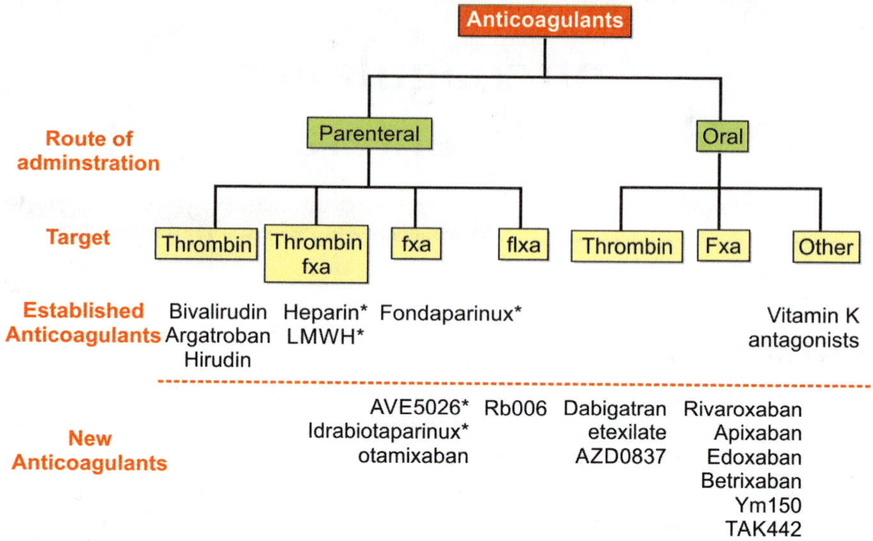

LMWH, low molecular weight heparin.

Fig. 1: Classification of anticoagulants[4]

*Indirectly inhibit coagulation by interacting with antithrombin.

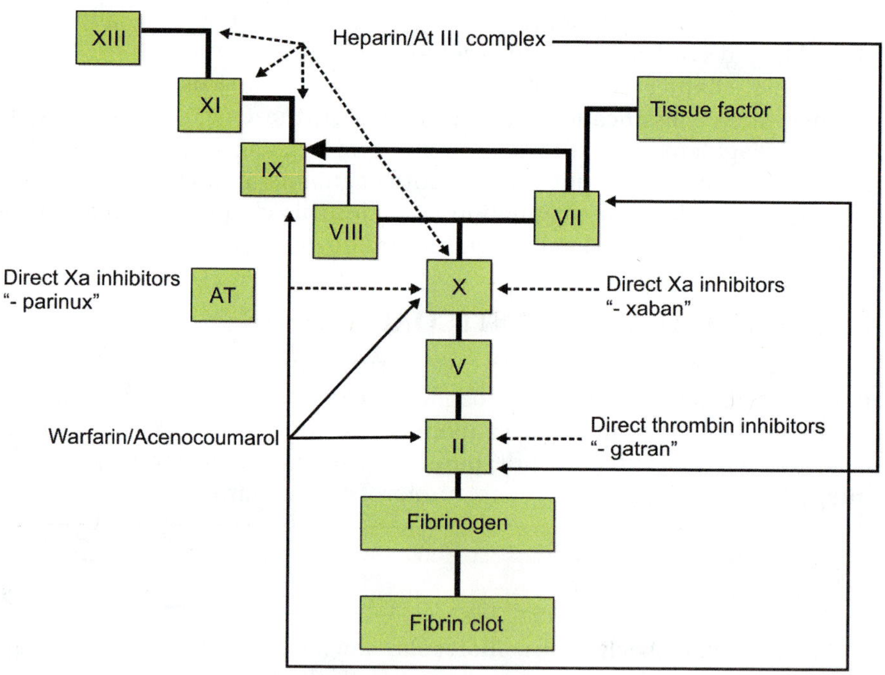

Fig. 2: Sites of action of various anticoagulants[7]

The cornerstone of anticoagulation therapy in conditions such as VTE, traditionally involves two overlapping steps: (i) initial treatment with a rapid-acting parenteral anticoagulant such as LMWH for at least 5 days and

(ii) subsequent overlapping with VKA treatment. Parenteral anticoagulant administration is stopped once VKA therapy is stable and therapeutic, as indicated by the international normalized ratio.[6]

Sites of Action of Anticoagulants in Coagulation Cascade

The sites of action of different classes of anticoagulant are shown in figure 2. Vitamin K antagonists inhibit the synthesis of vitamin K-dependent clotting factors II, VII, IX, and X. Newer agents, such as apixaban and rivaroxaban, act directly on factor Xa, while dabigatran acts directly on factor II.[7]

> Anticoagulants prevent thrombosis by interfering with the coagulation cascade.

FEATURES OF AN IDEAL ANTICOAGULANT

The properties of an ideal anticoagulant are summarized in table 1.[8]

Oral and Parenteral Anticoagulants in the Pipeline[9]

The issues and limitations associated with existing anticoagulants have driven the search for an ideal anticoagulant. These newer agents are aimed at targeting specific steps in the coagulation cascade directly. Anticoagulants in the developmental pipeline include:

> An ideal anticoagulant is one that has a rapid onset of action with a predictable pharmacokinetic and coagulation response.

- Newer LMWHs (adomiparin)
- Ultra LMWHs (semuloparin, RO-14)

Table 1: Desired properties of an ideal anticoagulant

Characteristics	Consequences
Rapid onset of action	No need for overlap with parenteral anticoagulants; simplified management in case of a hemorrhagic event or need for an intervention and minimizes need for an antidote
Predictable pharmacokinetics	Simplified dosing regimens
Predictable anticoagulant response	Fixed dose, no need for coagulation monitoring and dose adjustment
Oral availability	New indications
No CYP2C9 or VCOR1 metabolism	Lack of food interactions, few if any drug interactions
Availability of a safe antidote	Provide rapid reversal in case of a hemorrhagic event or need for an intervention
No off-target effects, such as hepatoxicity	No need for monitoring
Reasonable cost	Improved access, favors use for new indications

- Inhibitors of activated factor II (dabigatran, AZD0837)
- Inhibitors of activated factor X (rivaroxaban, apixaban, edoxaban, and betrixaban)
- Inhibitors of activated factor IX (REG1, 2)
- Inhibitors of activated factor XI (antisense oligonucleotides, BMS 262084, clavatadine A)
- Inhibitors of activated factor VII/tissue factor (tifacogin, PCI 274836, and BMS 593214)
- Inhibitors of activated factor V (recomodulin and solulin)
- Inhibitors of activated factor VIII (TB402)
- Dual thrombin/factor X inhibitors (EP21709, tanogitran)
- Newer VKAs (tecarfarin).

The sites of action of these newer oral and parenteral novel anticoagulants under development are shown in figure 3.

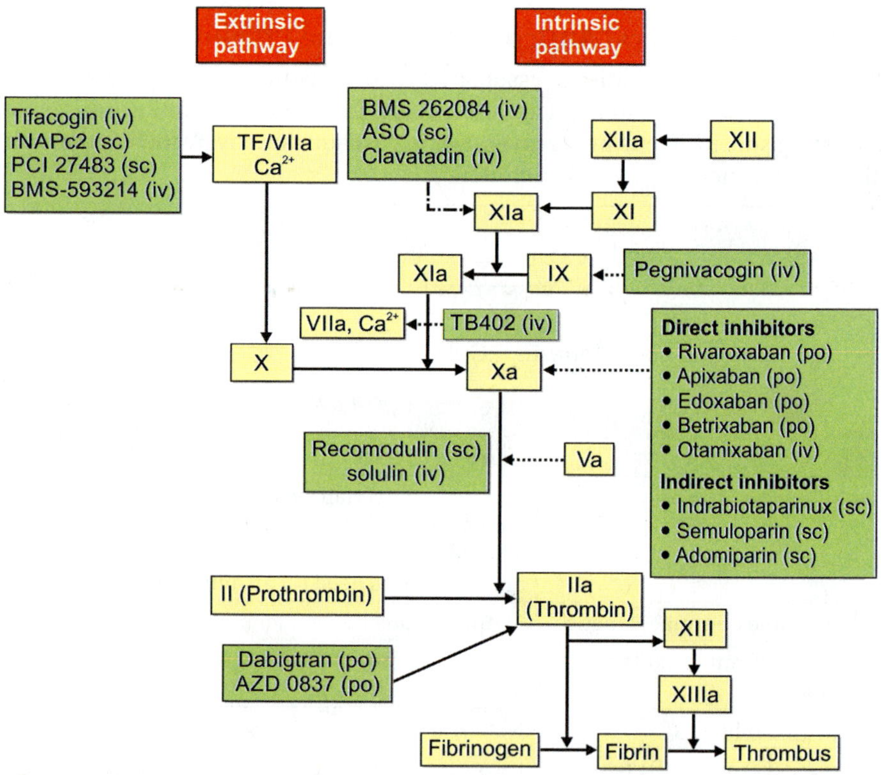

PO, oral; IV, intravenous; SC, subcutaneous; rNAPc2, recombinant nematode anticoagulant protein; ASO, antisense oligonucleotides.

Fig. 3: Target sites of novel anticoagulants (in green) in the coagulation cascade (in yellow), along with their routes of administration (in brackets)[9]

KEY POINTS

- Anticoagulants are widely used for the primary as well as secondary prevention of thromboembolic events
- Anticoagulants can be broadly classified as parenteral and oral anticoagulants
- Heparins and VKAs have been used conventionally over many years for clinical anticoagulation therapy
- Newer anticoagulants with specific target sites in the coagulation cascade have been developed
- Certain new molecules are also in the development pipeline.

REFERENCES

1. Gomez-Outes A, Luisa Suarez-Gea M, Calvo-Rojas G, Lecumberri R, Rocha E, Pozo-Hernández C, et al. Discovery of anticoagulant drugs: a historical perspective. Curr Drug Discov Technol. 2012;9:83-104.
2. Hawes EM, Viera AJ. Anticoagulation: indications and risk classification schemes. FP Essent. 2014;422:11-17.
3. Keeling D, Baglin T, Tait C, Watson H, Perry D, Baglin C, et al. Guidelines on oral anticoagulation with warfarin—fourth edition. Br J Haematol. 2011;154:311-24.
4. Eikelboom JW, Weitz JI. New anticoagulants. Circulation. 2010;121:1523-32.
5. Garcia D, Libby E, Crowther MA. The new oral anticoagulants. Blood. 2010;115:15-20.
6. Yeh C, Gross P, Weitz J. Evolving use of new oral anticoagulants for treatment of venous thromboembolism. Blood. 2014;124:1020-8.
7. Anticoagulant agents. JAPI. 2014;62:10-8.
8. Manoria P, Manoria PC. Newer antithrombotics and anticoagulants. Medicine Update. 2010;20:346-50.
9. Aditya S. Oral and parenteral anticoagulants: new kids on the block. J Postgrad Med. 2012;58:275-85.

3

Indications of Anticoagulation Therapy

Yogendra Singh

INTRODUCTION

Anticoagulants are widely prescribed for the prevention and management of thromboembolic disorders and for stroke prevention in patients with atrial fibrillation.[1] In this chapter, entitled the common as well as uncommon indications of vitamin K antagonists (VKAs) are discussed. Furthermore, the current indications of newer oral anticoagulants are also discussed.

CURRENT INDICATIONS OF VITAMIN K ANTAGONISTS AND THE RECOMMENDED INTENSITY OF ANTICOAGULATION

Oral anticoagulants are indicated in the prevention of venous thromboembolism; treatment of deep vein thrombosis; and prevention of thromboembolic events in myocardial infarction, prosthetic heart valves, atrial fibrillation, and valvular heart disease.[2] Apart from stroke prevention, anticoagulants are also indicated in certain noncardiac indications in neurology, where the risk of thromboembolism is high. These include intracranial malignancy, spinal cord injury, antiphospholipid syndrome, and cerebral venous sinus thrombosis.[3]

The 2012 American College of Chest Physicians (ACCP) recommendations for the use of VKAs are summarized in table 1.[4-8]

CURRENT INDICATIONS OF NEWER ORAL ANTICOAGULANTS

The era of new oral anticoagulants began with the approval of dabigatran by Food and Drug Administration in 2010. This was followed by the approval of rivaroxaban and apixaban in 2011 and 2012, respectively.[9] Current indications of these newer oral anticoagulants, based on their approval, have been summarized in table 2.

Table 1: Vitamin K antagonists^: Current indications and intensity

Indication (Recommendation grade as per ACCP)	DVT of the leg or PE*			
	First episode (1B)	**Cancer (1B)**	**Antiphospholipid antibody (2B)**	**Second episode (1B)**
Target INR (range)	2.5 (2.0 to 3.0)	2.5 (2.0 to 3.0)	2.5 (2.0 to 3.0)	2.5 (2.0 to 3.0)
Duration of therapy (ACCP recommendation grade)	In patients with the first episode of proximal DVT or PE due to surgery: • Recommended for 3 months over short-term use (1B), longer use (1B), or extended therapy duration (1B) In patients with the first episode of proximal DVT or PE due to a reversible risk factor: • Preferred for 3 months over short-term use (1B), longer use (1B), or extended therapy duration (1B or 2B, depending on bleeding risk†) In patients with the first episode of distal DVT (due to surgery or a reversible risk factor): • Preferred for 3 months over short-term use (2C), longer use (1B), or extended therapy duration (1B) In patients with the first episode of idiopathic proximal DVT or PE: • Low or moderate bleeding risk†: extended use recommended over 3 months (2B); high bleeding risk†: recommended for 3 months, over extended use (1B for DVT; 1B for PE) In patients with the first episode of idiopathic distal DVT: • Recommended for 3 months over extended use (1B or 2B, depending on bleeding risk†)	In patients with active cancer and PE: • Low-molecular-weight heparin preferred over VKA; extended use recommended (1B or 2B, depending on bleeding risk†)	In patients with antiphospholipid antibody and history of arterial or venous thrombosis: • Recommended for extended duration, with target INR of 2.5 over higher range of 3.0 to 4.5 (2B)	In patients with two episodes of unprovoked DVT or PE: • Low (1B) or moderate bleeding risk†: extended therapy (2B) • High bleeding risk†: 3 months (2B)

Table 1: Vitamin K antagonists^: Current indications and intensity (continued)

Indication (Recommendation grade as per ACCP)	Atrial fibrillation or flutter			
	Intermediate†-to-high§ risk of stroke‖ (1B)	**Elective cardio version (1B)**	**Antiphospholipid antibody (2B)**	**After stent placement and when risk of stroke is high (2C)**
Target INR (range)	2.5 (2.0 to 3.0)	2.5 (2.0 to 3.0)	2.5 (2.0 to 3.0)	2.5 (2.0 to 3.0)
Duration of therapy (Recommendation grade as per ACCP)	Indefnite VKA therapy	VKAs started 3 weeks before if scheduled and for 4 weeks after conversion (1B/2C)	Indefinite VKA therapy	• In patients with bare-metal stent (1 month) and drug-eluting stent (3–6 months), VKA is used as triple therapy with clopidogrel and aspirin (2C) • After initial triple therapy, continue VKA and a single antiplatelet agent until 12 months after stent placement (2C) • After 12 months: VKA alone (2C)
Indication (Recommendation grade as per ACCP)	**Coronary heart disease**			
	High-risk patients with myocardial infarction without a stent¶ (1B)		**High-risk patients with myocardial infarction and after stent placement¶ (2C)**	
Target INR (range)	2.5 (2.0 to 3.0) with low-dose aspirin (75–100 mg daily)		2.5 (2.0 to 3.0)	
Duration of therapy (Recommendation grade as per ACCP)	3 months of VKA therapy		• In patients with bare-metal stent: triple therapy with VKA, low-dose aspirin, and clopidogrel in month 1; combination of VKA with single antiplatelet agent in months 2 and 3 • In patients with drug-eluting stent: triple therapy with VKA, low-dose aspirin, and clopidogrel for 3 to 6 months	

Continued

Continued

Table 1: Vitamin K antagonists^: Current indications and intensity (continued)

Indication (Recommendation grade as per ACCP)	Valvular heart disease		
	Rheumatic mitral valve disease (1A if patient has atrial fibrillation or a history of systemic embolism; 1A if patient has history of atrial thrombus; 2C if patient has normal sinus rhythm and atrial diameter >55 mm)	**Mechanical prosthetic heart valves [aortic position (2C over low-range INR and 1B over highrange INR); mitral position (2C over low-range INR)]**	**Bioprosthetic valves in the mitral position (2C)**
Target INR (range)	2.5 (2.0 to 3.0)	Bileaflet or tilting-disk valves: 2.5 (2.0 to 3.0) in the aortic position, and 3.0 (2.5 to 3.5) in the mitral position	2.5 (2.0 to 3.0)
Duration of therapy (Recommendation grade as per ACCP)	Long-term VKA therapy	• Long-term VKA therapy • Recommended to use aspirin, 50 to 100 mg daily, with mechanical aortic or mitral valve and low bleeding risk	3 months of VKA therapy after insertion

Continued

Continued

Table 1: Vitamin K antagonists^: Current indications and intensity (continued)

Indication (Recommendation grade as per ACCP)	Prevention of venous thromboembolism in orthopedic surgery	
	Elective total hip or knee replacement and hip fracture surgery (1B)	**Nil**
Target INR (range)	2.5 (2.0 to 3.0)	**Nil**
Elective total hip or knee replacement and hip fracture surgery (1B)	• VKA therapy for a minimum of 10 to 14 days (1B) • VKA therapy for 35 days for major orthopedic surgery (2B)	VKAs are second-line agents to low-molecular-weight heparin for total hip or total knee arthroplasty (2C)

ACCP, American College of Chest Physicians; CHADS2, congestive heart failure, hypertension, age ≥75 years, diabetes mellitus, prior ischemic stroke, or transient ischemic attack (doubled); DVT, Deep venous thrombosis; INR, International normalized ratio; PE, Pulmonary embolism; VKA, vitamin K antagonists.

NOTE: Grade 1 recommendations are strong recommendations that can be applied to most patients; grade 2 recommendations are weaker recommendations. Grade A recommendations are supported by high-quality evidence, grade B recommendations are based on randomized clinical trials with methodological flaws or inconsistent results, and grade C recommendations are based on weaker evidence.

*Recommendation to start warfarin on the first day of treatment with a parenteral anticoagulant (unfractionated or low-molecular-weight heparin, or fondaparinux [Arixtra]); 1B.

†Risk factors that increase a patient's bleeding risk include advanced age, active gastric or duodenal ulcer, recent gastrointestinal bleeding, history of stroke, myocardial infarction, diabetes, and several laboratory abnormalities (e.g., elevated creatinine level, low platelet count, low hematocrit level).

‡Defined as a CHADS2 score of 1.

§Defined as a CHADS2 score of 2 or greater.

||Of note, in patients with a CHADS2 score of 0, aspirin (75 to 325 mg daily) is recommended as an option; 2B.

¶Patients with large anterior wall myocardial infarction who have left ventricular thrombus or who are at high risk of left ventricular thrombus (ejection fraction <40 percent or anteroapical wall motion abnormality); 1B.

^Vitamin K antagonists: Warfarin

Table 2: Current indications of newer oral anticoagulants

New anticoagulant	Approval
Dabigatran[4]	• To reduce the risk of stroke and systemic embolism in patients with non-valvular atrial fibrillation • To treat DVT and PE in patients who have been treated with a parenteral anticoagulant for 5–10 days • To reduce the risk of recurrence of DVT and PE in patients who have been previously treated • To prevent DVT and PE in patients who have undergone hip replacement surgery
Rivaroxaban[5]	• To reduce the risk of stroke and systemic embolism in patients who have nonvalvular atrial fibrillation • To treat DVT and PE, and for the reduction in the risk of recurrence of DVT and of PE • To prevent DVT and subsequent PE in patients undergoing knee or hip replacement surgery
Apixaban[6]	• To reduce the risk of stroke and systemic embolism in patients with nonvalvular atrial fibrillation • To prevent DVT, which may lead to PE, in patients who have undergone hip or knee replacement surgery • To treat DVT and PE, and for the reduction in the risk of recurrent DVT and PE following initial therapy

DVT: Deep vein thrombosis; PE: Pulmonary embolism.

KEY POINTS

- Anticoagulants are required in a range of clinical conditions, for the prophylaxis and treatment of thromboembolic events
- Vitamin K antagonists have been recommended in indications such as stroke prevention in atrial fibrillation, prevention and treatment of DVT and pulmonary embolism, and valvular and nonvalvular heart disease
- Newer oral anticoagulants have limited indications and are indicated in nonvalvular atrial fibrillation and in the prevention and treatment of VTE after orthopedic surgery.

REFERENCES

1. Hirsh J, Dalen GE, Anderson DR, Poller L, Bussey H, Ansell J, et al. Oral anticoagulants: Mechanism of action, clinical effectiveness, and optimal therapeutic range. Chest. 2001;119(Suppl 1):8S-21S.
2. Hirsh J, Fuster V. Guide to anticoagulant therapy. Part 2: Oral anticoagulants. Circulation. 1994;89(3):1469-80.
3. Marshall AL, Connors JM. Anticoagulation for noncardiac indications in neurologic patients: Comparative use of non-vitamin k oral anticoagulants, low-molecular-weight heparins and warfarin. Curr Treat Options Neurol. 2014;16(9):309.

4. Kearon C, Akl EA, Comerota AJ, Prandoni P, Bounameaux H, Goldhaber SZ, et al. Antithrombotic therapy for VTE disease. Antithrombotic therapy and prevention of thrombosis, 9th ed. American College of Chest Physicians Evidence-Based Clinical Practice Guidelines. Chest. 2012;141(2 Suppl): e419S-94S.
5. You JJ, Singer DE, Howard PA, Lane DA, Eckman MH, Fang MC, et al. Antithrombotic therapy for atrial fibrillation. Antithrombotic Therapy and Prevention of Thrombosis, 9th ed: American College of Chest Physicians Evidence-Based Clinical Practice Guidelines. Chest. 2012;141(2 Suppl):e531S-75S.
6. Whitlock RP, Sun JC, Fremes SE, Rubens FD, Teoh KH; American College of Chest Physicians. Antithrombotic and thrombolytic therapy for valvular disease. Antithrombotic Therapy and Prevention of Thrombosis, 9th ed. American College of Chest Physicians Evidence-Based Clinical Practice Guidelines. Chest. 2012;141(2 Suppl):e576S-600S.
7. Vandvik PO, Lincoff AM, Gore JM, Gutterman DD, Sonnenberg FA, Alonso-Coello P, et al. Primary and secondary prevention of cardiovascular disease: Antithrombotic Therapy and Prevention of Thrombosis, 9th ed. American College of Chest Physicians Evidence-Based Clinical Practice Guidelines. Chest. 2012;141(2 Suppl):e637S-68S.
8. Falck-Ytter Y, Francis CW, Johanson NA, Curley C, Dahl OE, Schulman S, et al. Prevention of VTE in orthopedic surgery patients. Antithrombotic Therapy and Prevention of Thrombosis, 9th ed. American College of Chest Physicians Evidence-Based Clinical Practice Guidelines. Chest. 2012;141(2 Suppl):e278S-325S.
9. Wigle P, Hein B, Bloomfield HE, Tubb M, Doherty M. Updated guidelines on outpatient anticoagulation. Am Fam Physician. 2013;87(8):556-66.
10. Dabigatran (Prescribing Information) 2015. [online] Available from: http://www.accessdata.fda.gov/drugsatfda_docs/label/2015/022512s028lbl.pdf. [Accessed January, 2017].
11. Rivaroxaban [Prescribing Information] 2015. [online] Available from: http://www.accessdata.fda.gov/drugsatfda_docs/label/2015/022406s012lbl.pdf. Accessed on: 01 August 2016.
12. Apixaban [Prescribing Information] 2015. Available from: http://www.accessdata.fda.gov/drugsatfda_docs/label/2015/202155s011lbl.pdf. [Accessed January, 2017].

4

Oral Anticoagulants: From Discovery to Clinical Practice

K Damodara Rao Kodem, Mrinal K Das

INTRODUCTION TO ORAL ANTICOAGULANTS

Today there is a need for chronic anticoagulation therapy, due to the rising prevalence of atrial fibrillation (AF), artificial heart valves, and malignancy among the aging population. Anticoagulant treatment is indicated for the treatment and prevention of arterial and venous thromboembolic disorders, such as stroke, pulmonary embolism (PE), venous thromboembolism (VTE), and acute coronary syndrome. Patients with AF have a fivefold higher risk of stroke-related fatality or disability. Oral anticoagulants have been mainly indicated for stroke prevention in AF patients. There is also a significant need for anticoagulation therapy in patients undergoing orthopedic surgeries (hip or knee replacement), due to a higher risk of PE or VTE.[1]

In the past two decades, the interest in antithrombotic compounds with a distinct mode of action on the coagulation pathway has lead to the approval of anticoagulants such as low molecular weight heparins, indirect factor Xa inhibitors, and direct thrombin inhibitors. However, factors such as higher cost of therapy and the need for parenteral administration have resulted in oral vitamin K antagonists being the only alternative anticoagulant for patients requiring chronic anticoagulation therapy.[2] The commonly used vitamin K antagonists in clinical practice are coumarin preparations.[3]

In this chapter, we will discuss the history of coumarin derivatives: from their discovery to their use as anticoagulants in clinical practice.

> Vitamin K antagonists are among the most commonly used anticoagulants in clinical practice.

HISTORY OF TWO DISCOVERIES THAT LED TO THE AVAILABILITY OF CLINICAL ANTICOAGULANTS

Two different lines of research in the 1920s and 1930s led to the discovery of vitamin K and its antagonists.[4]

Discovery of Vitamin K[5]

Between 1928 and 1930, unexpected symptoms of hemorrhage and delayed coagulation in chicks being reared for metabolic studies prompted Henrik Carl Peter Dam and his coworkers to further investigate the cause. During

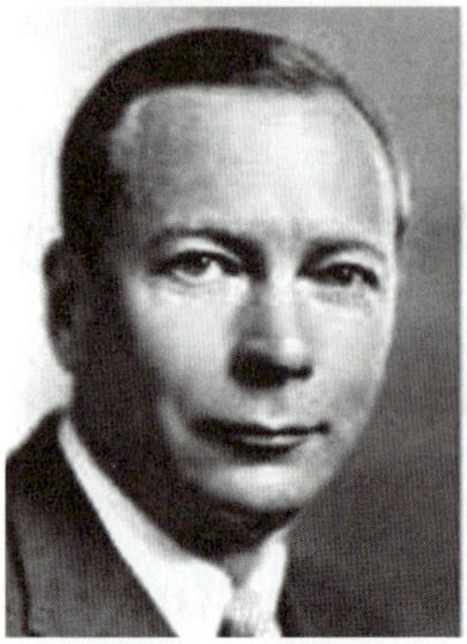
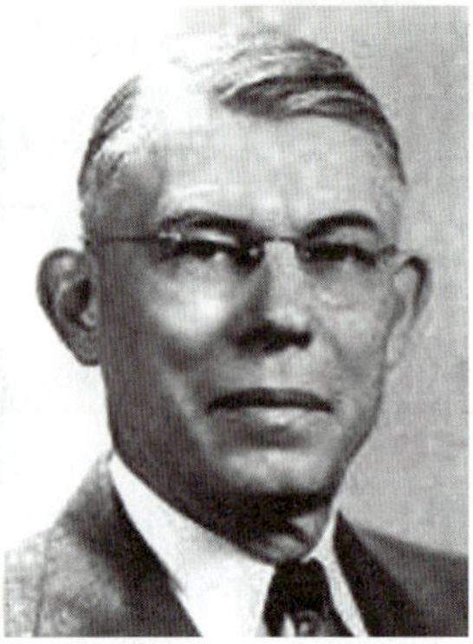

Henrik Carl Peter Dam Edward Adelbert Doisy

the course of the investigation, they found that an unrecognized factor in the diet of the chicks was able to prevent hemorrhagic symptoms. In 1935, this factor was characterized as a new fat-soluble vitamin and designated vitamin K [the letter K stands for Koagulation (coagulation)]. Edward Adelbert Doisy elucidated the chemical structure of vitamin K over the next 10 years, and reported its method of synthesis.[4]

In 1943, Henrik Dam and Edward Doisy jointly won the Nobel Prize for their contributions to the understanding of blood clotting, especially the role of vitamin K.

Discovery of Coumarin Anticoagulants[6,7]

The Epidemic of Sweet Clover Disease

Between 1920 and 1922, the cattle population of the Canadian and North American prairies faced a fatal epidemic of generalized bleeding diathesis. The hemorrhagic disease that manifested within 15 days of ingestion of moldy sweet clover hay, and led to death within 30–50 days, was termed sweet clover disease. Frank W Schofield, a Canadian pathologist, proved that the causative

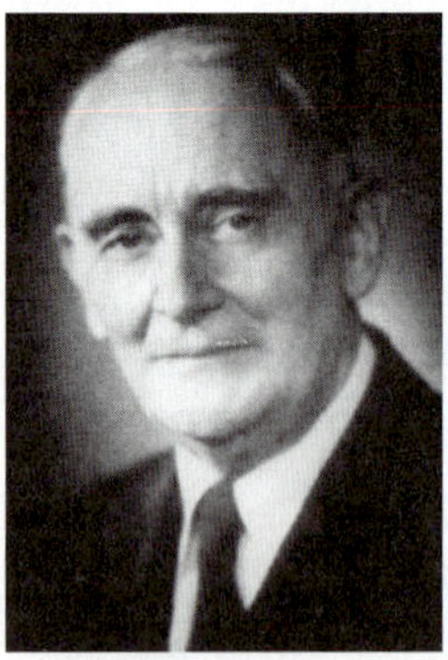

Frank W Schofield

factor was a substance found in moldy sweet clover hay. He further proved that the disease condition was potentially reversible if the offending hay was removed from the diet or the animals transfused with fresh blood.

Isolation of Anticoagulant from the Rotten Clover

Between 1933 and 1939, Karl Paul Link and his colleagues attempted to isolate the anticoagulant present in the rotten clover. In 1939, they were finally able to crystallize the substance, which was proven to be dicoumarol [3,3′-methylene-bis(4-hydroxycoumarin)], a product formed due to the oxidation of naturally occurring coumarin in sweet clover. Consequently, they demonstrated that vitamin K could counter the anticoagulant action of dicoumarol.

From Test Tube to Rat Poison

In 1945, Link dwelled upon the idea of using the hemorrhagic property of a coumarin derivative as a rodenticide. The slow-acting characteristics of dicoumarol led Link and his colleagues to test several variations of naturally occurring coumarin in search of a fast-acting compound. Warfarin was the product of this effort, and was promoted as a rodenticide in 1948.[6]

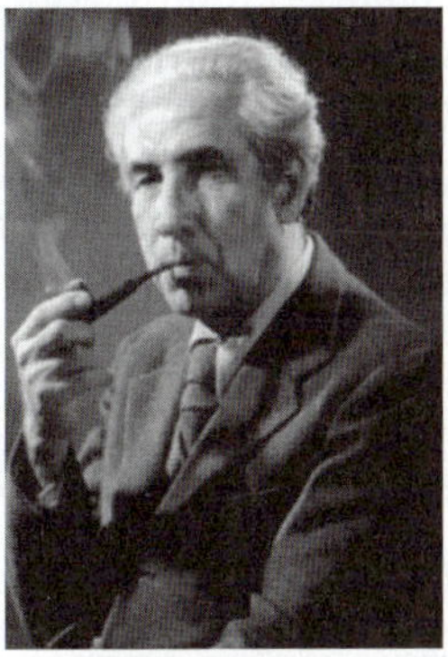

Karl Paul Link

From Rat Poison to Clinical Use

The success of warfarin as a rodenticide, and its apparent advantages over heparin and dicoumarol, coupled with its high water solubility and oral bioavailability, supported its use in clinical conditions. Warfarin was not used frequently until 1955, when it was administered to President Dwight D Eisenhower following a myocardial infarction. This led to the widespread prescription of the drug.[6] Earlier in 1941, the Mayo Clinic had reported the successful use of dicoumarol in the prophylaxis of deep-vein thrombosis after surgery.[8]

This is the fascinating journey of coumarin anticoagulant, which went from being a test tube discovery to being promoted as a rat poison and eventually becoming a wonder drug for the prevention and treatment of thromboembolic disorders.

YET ANOTHER BREAKTHROUGH: THE DEVELOPMENT OF ACENOCOUMAROL

In an effort to develop the perfect anticoagulant, Stoll and Litvan (Ciba Geigy) developed Nicoumalone (acenocoumarol) in 1953. Acenocoumarol found clinical use in Europe in 1955 followed by the United States in 1956.[8]

Some of the features of acenocoumarol that established its superiority over other anticoagulants include:[3]

- Rapid onset of action
- Long-term anticoagulation effect lasting 15–20 hours
- Superior anticoagulation stability compared to warfarin
- Rapid reversal of anticoagulant action with relatively small doses of vitamin K1
- Reduced dependence on CYP2C9 enzyme than on warfarin for metabolism.

> Acenocoumarol is used in the treatment of various thromboembolic disorders and has well-documented safety and efficacy.

The clinical use of oral anticoagulants has come a long way since their discovery in 1943. Following over 50 years of clinical experience and numerous clinical studies, acenocoumarol could be considered close to an ideal oral anticoagulant. The well-documented safety and efficacy of acenocoumarol, and its efficacy and superiority over warfarin in maintaining international normalized ration stability within the therapeutic range, have made it a drug of choice in the treatment of various thromboembolic disorders.[8] It also finds a mention in several reputed medical books, such as:

Goodman and Gilman's The Pharmacological basis of Therapeutics, 12th Edition
"Acenocoumarol has a short half-life (10–24 hours), more rapid effect on the prothrombin time and short duration of action (2 days)."
Martindale: The Extra Pharmacopoeia, 36th Edition
"Acenocoumarol is used in the management of thromboembolic disorders."
Essentials of Pharmacology by KD Tripathi
"Acenocoumarol is considered among the suitable and well tolerated anticoagulants."
Postgraduate Haematolog, 6th Edition
"Studies with acenocoumarol have demonstrated better safety profile in patients with venous thromboembolism."

KEY POINTS

- Efforts to identify the hemorrhagic factor responsible for sweet clover disease led to the discovery of coumarin anticoagulants
- Coumarin derivatives were initially promoted as rodenticides, but later developed for use in clinical therapeutics
- The well-documented safety and efficacy of acenocoumarol make it a favorable option in oral anticoagulant therapy.

REFERENCES

1. Miesbach W, Seifried E. New direct oral anticoagulants-current therapeutic options and treatment recommendations for bleeding complications. Thromb Haemost. 2012;108(4):625-32.
2. Garcia D, Libby E, Crowther MA. The new oral anticoagulants. Blood. 2010;115(1):15-20.
3. Trailokya A, Hiremath JS, Sawhney J, Mishra YK, Kanhere V, Srinivasa R, et al. Acenocoumarol: A review of anticoagulant efficacy and safety. J Assoc Physicians India. 2016;64(2):88-93.
4. Hemker HC, Frank HL. The mechanism of action of oral anticoagulants and its consequences for the practice of oral anticoagulation. Haemostasis. 1985;15(4):263-70.
5. Dam H. (1946). The discovery of vitamin K, its biological functions and therapeutical application. Nobel Lecture. [online] Available from: http://www.nobelprize.org/nobel_prizes/medicine/laureates/1943/dam-lecture.pdf. [Accessed January, 2016].
6. Wardrop D, Keeling D. The story of the discovery of heparin and warfarin. Br J Haematol. 2008;141(6):757-63.
7. Karatzas NB. Coumarins, a class of drugs with a unique contribution to medicine: the tale of their discovery. Hellenic J Cardiol. 2014;55(2):89-91.
8. Trailokya A. Acenocoumarol in thromoembolic disorders. Cardiovasc Pharm Open Access. 2015;4(4):157.

5

Vitamin K Antagonists in Thromboembolic Disorders

B Kesavamoorthy, Jagdish Hiremath

INTRODUCTION

Anticoagulant treatment has been indicated for the treatment and prevention of thromboembolic disorders. vitamin K antagonists (VKAs) are the most widely used oral anticoagulants worldwide.[1] This chapter, entitled "Vitamin K Antagonists in Thromboembolic Disorders", touches upon the thromboembolic disorder scenario in India. It further discusses the mode of action of VKAs, including acenocoumarol; the pharmacokinetic aspects of VKAs; and also gives a comparative analysis of acenocoumarol and warfarin in the treatment of thromboembolism.

THROMBOEMBOLIC DISORDERS: INDIAN SCENARIO

The term venous thromboembolism (VTE) includes deep vein thrombosis (DVT) and pulmonary embolism (PE). More than 50% of patients undergoing surgical procedures, especially those involving the hip and knee, and around 10–40% of patients undergoing abdominal or thoracic surgery, are prone to VTE. Deep vein thrombosis is often asymptomatic and may develop into unrecognized PE.[1]

Venous and arterial thromboembolic diseases are still the most common cause of morbidity and mortality in developed countries, and their incidence has seen a dramatic rise in developing countries as well.[1]

The popular notion that VTE is less prevalent in the Indian population compared with the Western population has been disproved in recent studies.[2] Table 1 provides an overview of some of the studies conducted in India with respect to VTE incidence.

The provision of appropriate VTE prophylaxis remains inadequate in premier institutes in India, despite the availability of scientific evidence supporting its importance. Hence, there is a need for the implementation of hospital-wide strategies for proper patient risk assessment and the subsequent initiation of prophylactic measures.[2]

> Around 80% of all deep vein thrombosis cases are asymptomatic.[2] Of all the fatal pulmonary embolism cases, less than half are detected prior to death.[2]

Table 1: Indian studies on venous thromboembolism incidence[2]

Author/type of study	Study population	Study outcome
Prospective observational study (smart study group)[3]	Asian patients (2,420 patients) undergoing major orthopedic surgery without thromboprophylaxis	Symptomatic VTE in 2.3% patients and sudden death in 1.2% patients
Prospective registry on venous thromboembolic events study[4]	Total 3,526 patients with symptomatic DVT from 19 countries; 667 were from India	DVT was found proximally and in the calf in 54% of Indian patients; comparable to Western data
Prospective study (Sharma et al.)[5]	112 patients who underwent surgery for fractures around hip joint	19.6% incidence of DVT
Multicentric study (Bhan et al.)[6]	180 patients undergoing orthopedic surgery	23.34% of DVT in the nonprophylaxis group compared to nil in the mechanical prophylaxis group
Retrospective study, CMC Vellore from 1996–2005 (Lee et al.)[7]	Hospitalized patients diagnosed with VTE between 1996 and 2005	• Confirmed DVT cases 17.46 per 10,000 admissions; 64% being nonsurgical, nontrauma patients • PE diagnosed in 14.9% of the study patients • Mortality rate in patients with confirmed PE was 13.5%
Pandey et al.[8]	117 hospitalized patients	The risk of DVT and PE was highest in 75% of the patients admitted to the medicine ward and medicine ICU. DVT prophylaxis within first two days of admission was just 12.5%
Shead et al.[9]	50 South Indian patients above 50 years of age	28% incidence of postoperative DVT
The ENDORSE global epidemiological study[10]	68,183 hospitalized patients across 32 countries; 2,058 patients were from India	54% of hospitalized (45% medical and 61% surgical) Indian patients had risk factor for VTE
Kakkar and Vasishta[11]	1,000 medical autopsies	Overall incidence of PE in medical autopsies (fatal, contributory, and incidental groups) was 15.9%; PE incidence was 79.87% in the younger population

DVT, deep vein thrombosis; PE, pulmonary embolism; ICU, intensive care unit; VTE, venous thromboembolism.

Vitamin K Antagonists: Mode of Action

Vitamin K antagonists have been frequently indicated for preventing various thromboembolic disorders, such as DVT, PE, stroke prevention in valvular/nonvalvular heart disease, and acute coronary syndrome.[1]

Mechanism of Action of Vitamin K Antagonists

The formation of γ-carboxyglutamates (Gla) on the N-terminal regions of vitamin K-dependent proteins results from the post-translational vitamin K-dependent carboxylation of glutamic acid residues. The γ-carboxylation process permits the coagulation proteins to undergo a conformational change mediated by calcium ions, a step necessary for the complexing of these vitamin K-dependent proteins to their cofactors on phospholipids. The carboxylation of vitamin K-dependent coagulation proteins (prothrombin, factor VII, factor IX, and factor X) is catalyzed by a carboxylase that requires the reduced form of vitamin K (vitamin KH2), molecular oxygen, and carbon dioxide. During this reaction, vitamin KH2 is oxidized to vitamin K epoxide, which is recycled to vitamin K by vitamin K epoxide reductase, which in turn is reduced to vitamin KH2 by vitamin K reductase.[12]

Vitamin-K oral anticoagulants act by interfering with the cyclic conversion of vitamin K and its 2,3 epoxide (vitamin K epoxide). This results in a depletion of vitamin KH2, which in turn limits the γ-carboxylation of vitamin K-dependent coagulant factors. Consequently, there is hepatic production and secretion of partially carboxylated and decarboxylated proteins, and a reduction in the amount of Gla residues on the prothrombin molecule, resulting in reduced coagulant activity. A 30% reduction in coagulant activity has been seen with the reduction in number of Gla residues from a normal compliment of 10–13 to 9, while a 95% reduction ensues with a reduction of residues to less than 6.[12] The mechanism of action of VKAs is illustrated in figure 1.[13]

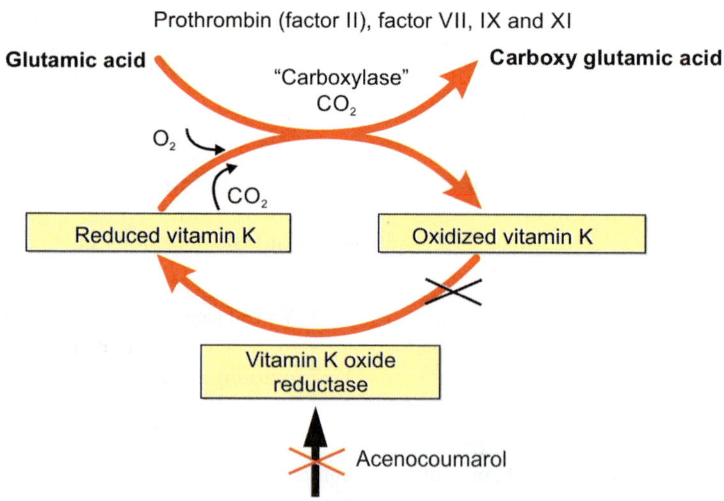

Fig. 1: Mechanism of action of vitamin K antagonist (acenocoumarol)[13]

A 30% reduction in coagulant activity is seen with the reduction in the number of Gla residues from a normal complement of 10–13 to 9, while a 95% reduction ensues with a reduction of residues to less than 6.

Structural Aspects of Acenocoumarol[13]

Acenocoumarol is one of the commonly used VKAs in clinical practice. It is a monocoumarin derivative with a racemic mixture of R (+) and S (–) enantiomers. The anticoagulant potency is found to be more in R (+) acenocoumarol compared to S (–) acenocoumarol. The presence of the nitro group in the para position of the phenyl ring renders it structurally different from warfarin (Fig. 2).[13]

Pharmacokinetics of Acenocoumarol[1]

The pharmacokinetic properties of acenocoumarol are summarized in table 2:

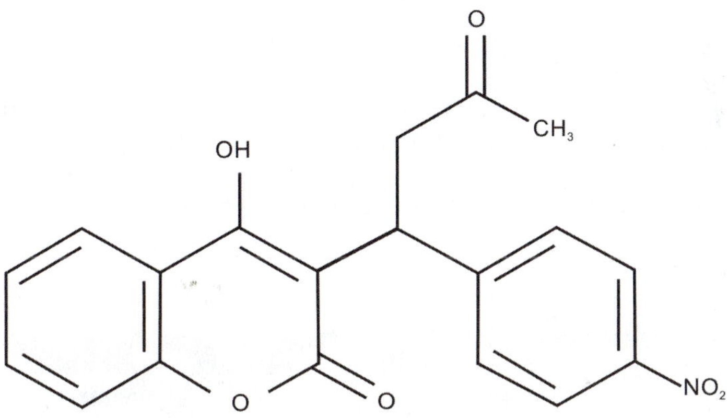

Fig. 2: Structure of acenocoumarol

Table 2: Pharmacokinetic properties of acenocoumarol

Absorption	Distribution	Metabolism	Elimination
• At least 60% of the administered dose of acenooumarol is systemically, available, indicating rapid absorption • Peak plasma concentrations are achieved within 1-3 h after a single dose of 10 mg	• Over 98% of acenocoumarol is protein-bound, essentially to albumin. The apparent volume of distribution is calculated to be 0.16–0.18 L/kg for the R(+) enantiomer and 0.22–0.34 L/kg for the S(–) enantiomer	• Acenocoumarol is extensively metabolized in humans, although the metabolites seem to be pharmacologically inactive	• It takes around 8–12 h for the elimination of the half-life of acenocoumarol from the plasma • 29% of the elimation is through faeces and 60% is through urine

COMPARATIVE ANALYSIS OF ACENOCOUMAROL AND WARFARIN

Acenocoumarol and warfarin are commonly used VKAs for the treatment and prevention of thromboembolic disorders. The rapid onset of action and the maintenance of therapy 15–20 hours after administration, offer acenocoumarol treatment great advantages over warfarin. The achievement of the therapeutic prothrombin level in just 36 hours after the initial dose of acenocoumarol and the requirement of relatively small doses of vitamin K1 for the reversal of anticoagulant activity add to its favorable characteristics.[1]

Additional benefits of acenocoumarol include:[1]

- Shorter half-life
- Better stability of prothrombin time
- Less dependence on CYP2C9 enzyme for metabolism.

Table 3 provides a pharmacokinetic comparison between acenocoumarol and warfarin.[14]

Clinical Studies Indicating Superior Efficacy of Acenocoumarol Over Warfarin

An observational study was conducted by Kulo et al. to evaluate the treatment quality with acenocoumarol versus warfarin among 120 patients with nonvalvular atrial fibrillation. It was reported that patients receiving acenocoumarol achieved better stability in terms of a longer time in the therapeutic range compared to those receiving warfarin (37.6 vs. 35.7%, $p = 0.05$) (Fig. 3).[15]

Table 3: Comparison of acenocoumarol and warfarin[14]

Properties	Warfarin	Acenocoumarol
Absorption	Rapid	Rapid
Bioavailability	99.4%	60%
Protein binding	Very high (99%)	Very high (98.7%)
Half-life	Distribution: 6–12 h Elimination: 20–60 h (mean 40 h)	8–11 h
Effect on PT	Within 24 h	15–20 h
Time to peak plasma concentration	4 h	1–3 h
Time to peak effect	72–96 h	36–48 h
Duration of action	2-5 days	48 h
Elimination	Renal 92%	Renal 60% Fecal 29%
Preparations available	1 mg, 2 mg, 3 mg, and 5 mg	0.5 mg, 1–4 mg tablets

PT, Prothrombin time.

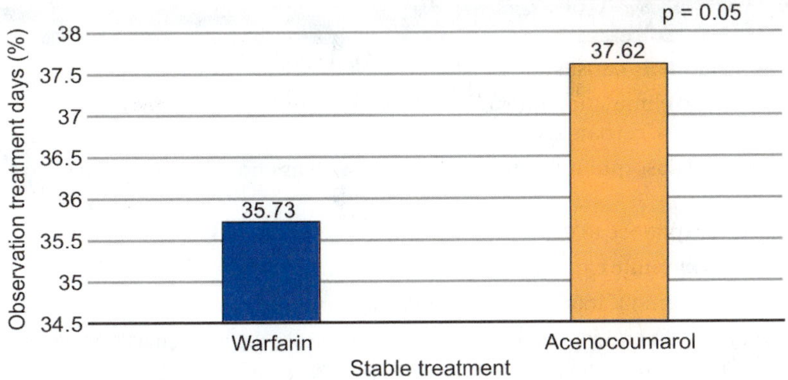

Fig. 3: Comparison of acenocoumarol and warfarin treatment stability

The Stroke Prevention Using Oral Thrombin Inhibitor in Atrial Fibrillation (SPORTIF III) study compared warfarin and acenocoumarol in 74 patients with atrial fibrillation. A better mean percentage of the international normalized ratio (INR) in the therapeutic range was observed in the acenocoumarol group compared to the warfarin group (56 vs. 49%, $p < 0.05$). Subtherapeutic INR incidence was higher with warfarin than with acenocoumarol (28 vs.19%, $p < 0.05$). Acenocoumarol was considered superior in terms of safety and efficacy, as it resulted in better INR stability at a much lower dose.[16]

In another study, 103 patients who switched to warfarin from acenocoumarol were compared within the same group to assess any improvement with respect to the quality and stability of treatment. The study concluded that warfarin did not improve the condition of the patients and that the difference between the two drugs could not be considered substantial as per clinical practice.[17]

Acenocoumarol in Warfarin Resistance

The inability to raise the INR to enter the therapeutic range at normal prescribed doses of the drug, or the failure to extend the prothrombin time, is described as warfarin resistance. It can be classified as either hereditary or acquired (such as poor compliance, drug interactions, and dietary interactions).[18] Some of the pharmacokinetic and pharmacodynamic causes of warfarin resistance are listed in box 1.[19]

Transitioning from Warfarin to Acenocoumarol

One of the approaches to the management of warfarin resistance involves the use of alternative anticoagulant therapy, which involves the use of medications such as acenocoumarol.[18]

Box 1: Causes of warfarin resistance[19]

Pharmacokinetic causes

- Enhanced elimination due to certain enzyme-inducing drugs, such as barbiturates, carbamazepine, and rifampin
- Impaired absorption due to medications such as cholestyramine and colestipol
- Poor compliance to the required dosage

Pharmacodynamic causes

- Excess vitamin K intake (health foods, dietary supplements, enteral feeds)
- Reduction in anticoagulant activity due to certain drugs such as estrogens, griseofulvin, 6-mercaptopurine, and haloperidol
- Hyperlipidemia (particularly hypercholesterolemia)
- Hypothyroidism
- Hereditary resistance (very rare)

In a published case study, an 80-year-old man with idiopathic iliofemoral vein thrombosis showed a reduced elevation in INR even after administration of increased doses of warfarin. However, the initiation of acenocoumarol after the discontinuation of warfarin treatment led to a considerable rise in INR, with sustained maintenance. The genotyping study suggested that the patient was predisposed to a high warfarin dose requirement; also, a rare mutation in *VKORC1* was suggested that influenced the warfarin dose, but not the acenocoumarol dose. This case study indicates that acenocoumarol use may be highly beneficial in patients with genetic warfarin resistance.[20]

According to a study, the transition factor between acenocoumarol and warfarin is 1.85. This indicates that the maintenance dose of warfarin is 1.85 times that of acenocoumarol.[21]

Long-Term Efficacy of Acenocoumarol

A Spanish study documented the 10-year experience of acenocoumarol use in 1,086 ambulatory patients with a mean age of 74 years. The most common indication for acenocoumarol usage in this cohort was atrial fibrillation. A total of 73% patients received acenocoumarol for atrial fibrillation. The study found that INR was in the therapeutic range (2.0–3.0) in 82.5% of patients. The overall bleeding and thrombotic event rates were low in the entire cohort (2.27/100 patients-years and 0.2/100 patients-years, respectively). The results showed that age and the therapeutic ranges of INR are not related to the increased risk of bleeding. The analysis also indicated the safety and efficacy of acenocoumarol use in the elderly population.[22]

In developing countries such as India, the medicinal use of long-term therapy is a huge health burden. According to an Indian study, the cost of acenocoumarol, including the cost of INR monitoring, is about 330 Indian rupees for a month. Hence, acenocoumarol can be an economically viable option for long-term anticoagulant therapy.[23]

KEY POINTS

- The incidence of venous thromboembolism is on the rise in India; it is comparable to that in the Western population
- The superior pharmacokinetic properties of acenocoumarol compared to warfarin make it a favorable option for anticoagulant therapy
- Acenocoumarol could be used as an alternative therapy in case of warfarin-resistance
- The long-term safety and efficacy of acenocoumarol, coupled with its cost-effectiveness, make it a preferred therapeutic option in patients requiring prolonged treatment, especially in those suffering from thromboembolic disorders.

REFERENCES

1. Trailokya A. Acenocoumarol in Thromboembolic Disorders. Cardiovasc Pharm Open Access. 2015;4:157.
2. Venous Thromboembolism-Indian Perspective. (2010). [online] Accessed from: www.Apiindia.Org/Pdf/Medicine_Update_2010/Cardiology_31.Pdf. [Accessed January, 2017].
3. Leizorovicz A, Turpie AG, Cohen AT, Wong L, Yoo MC, Dans A, et al. Epidemiology of venous thromboembolism in Asian Patients undergoing major orthopaedic surgery without thromboprophylaxis. The Smart Study. J Thromb Haemost. 2005;3(1):28-34.
4. Pinjala RK, Agarwal MB, Turpie AGG. For Prove Investigators. A Characterization of Patients With Symptomatic DVT In India. J. Thromb Haemost. 2005;3(Suppl 1):1043.
5. Sharma H, Maini L, Agarwal N, Upadhyay A, Vishwanath J, Dhaon BK. Incidence of deep vein thrombosis in patients with fracture around hip joint: a prospective study. Indian J Orthop. 2002;36(3):5.
6. Bhan S, Dhaon BK, Gulati Y, Aggarwal S. Deep venous thrombosis prophylaxis—A multicentric study. Indian J Orphtop. 2004;38(3):178-182.
7. Lee AD, Stephen E, Agarwal S, Premkumar P. Venous-thromboembolism in India. Eur J Vasc Endovasc Surg. 2009;37(4):482-5.
8. Pandey A, Patni N, Singh M, Randeep Guleria R. Assessment of risk and prophylaxis for deep vein thrombosis and pulmonary embolism in medically ill patients during their early days of hospital stay at a tertiary care centre in a developing country. Vasc Health Risk Manag. 2009;5:643-8.
9. Shead GV, Narayanan R. Incidence of post-operative venous thromboembolism in South India. Br J Surg. 1980;67(11):813-4.
10. Pinjala R. ENDORSE-India Investigators. Venous thromboembolism risk & prophylaxis in the acute hospital care setting (ENDORSE), a multinational cross-sectional study: results from the Indian subset data. Indian J Med Res. 2012;136(1):60-7.
11. Kakkar N, Vasishta RK. Pulmonary embolism in medical patients: an autopsy-based study. Clin Appl Thromb Hemost. 2008;14(2):159-67.
12. Hirsh J, Dalen JE, Deykin D, Poller L, Bussey H. Oral anticoagulants. Mechanism of action, clinical effectiveness, and optimal therapeutic range. Chest. 1992;102(4 Suppl):312-26.
13. Trailokya A, Hiremath JS, Sawhney J, Mishra YK, Kanhere V, Srinivasa R, et al. Acenocoumarol: A Review of Anticoagulant Efficacy and Safety. J Assoc Physicians India. 2016;64(2):88-93.
14. Anticoagulant agents. J Assoc Physicians India. 2014;62:10-8.
15. Kulo A, Kusturica J, Kapic E, Becić F, Rakanović-Todić M, Burnazović-Ristić L, et al. Better stability of acenocoumarol compared to warfarin treatment in one-year observational, clinical study in patients with nonvalvular atrial fibrillation. Med Glas (Zenica). 2011;8(1):9-14.
16. Lengyel M, SPORTIF-III Altanulmány Vizsgálói. [Warfarin or acenocoumarol is better in the anticoagulant treatment of chronic atrial fibrillation? Orv Hetil. 2004; 145(52):2619-21.

17. Barcellona D, Vannini ML, Fenu L, Balestrieri C, Marongiu F. Warfarin or acenocoumarol: which is better in the management of oral anticoagulants? Thromb Haemost. 1998;80(6): 899-902.
18. Lakshmi R, Anitha S, Anila KN, Roshni PR. Warfarin resistance-mechanisms and management. Int J Pharm Sci Res. 2012;3(2):353-57.
19. Parvizi R, Makhdami N, Dinparasti R. Warfarin resistance, a case report. J Cardiovasc Thorac Res. 2011;2(4):35-7.
20. Marusic S, Gojo-Tomic N, Franic M, Bozina N. Therapeutic efficacy of acenocoumarol in a warfarin-resistant patient with deep venous thrombosis: a case report. Eur J Clin Pharmacol. 2009;65(12):1265-6.
21. Van Leeuwen Y, Rosendaal F, Van Der Meer F. The relationship between maintenance dosages of three vitamin K antagonists: acenocoumarol, warfarin and phenprocoumon. Thromb Res. 2008;123(2):225-30.
22. Trullas-Vila J, Bisbe-Company J, Freitas-Ramírez A, Soler-Simon S, Bisbe-Company V, Roncero-Vidal JM, et al. Ten-year experience with acenocoumarol treatment in an ambulatory cohort of Spanish patients. J Thromb Thrombolysis. 2009;28(4):436-43.
23. Azim A, Baronia AK, Rao BP, Singh RK, Gurjar M, Singh N. Safety and cost-effectiveness of acitrom for DVT prophylaxis in critically ill patients requiring prolonged mechanical ventilation—A preliminary experience. J Anaesth Clin Pharmacol. 2010;26(3):360-62.

6

Tests for Monitoring Adequacy and Efficacy of Anticoagulation Therapy

Nazir I Juvale

INTRODUCTION

The therapeutic administration of oral anticoagulants (OACs) has been the cornerstone of the treatment and prevention of morbidity and mortality associated with arterial thrombosis, atrial fibrillation (AF), venous thromboembolism (VTE), and recurrent thrombosis.[1,2] Vitamin K antagonists (VKAs) constitute the most widely used OACs. Vast clinical validation and published evidence have proved the efficacy of VKAs, which are the mainstay of OAC therapy.[2] This chapter discusses various aspects related to monitoring the adequacy and efficacy of VKA therapy.

MONITORING ORAL ANTICOAGULATION WITH VITAMIN K ANTAGONISTS

The objective of long-term anticoagulation therapy, especially in AF and VTE, is the reduction of the lifetime risk of stroke and recurrent thrombosis. Hence, monitoring the effect of OAC therapy is of prime importance. Moreover, there exist a wide range of inter- and intra-patient differences in dose requirements. This may be due to several factors that interfere with VKA uptake and metabolism in the liver, such as certain foods, medications, and comorbidities. Hence, an individualized dose regimen, rather than a fixed low-dose regimen, is preferred for maintaining the desired international normalized ratio (INR) target.[1]

The primary goal of monitoring VKA therapy is the establishment of the appropriate dose of VKA at therapy initiation and subsequent maintenance doses, based on the level of anticoagulation achieved. Monitoring also ensures the prevention of adverse events such as over-coagulation and associated complications. Proper dose adjustments, aided by routine monitoring, help in avoiding adverse events well in time, and prevent recurrence.[2]

Monitoring Vitamin K Antagonists Therapy—Prothrombin Time/International Normalized Ratio

The prothrombin time (PT) test is the most commonly used test for monitoring VKA therapy. Prothrombin time corresponds to a reduction of vitamin K-dependent procoagulant clotting factors II, VII, and X to a rate proportional to their respective half-lives, by VKAs. Thus, it can be safely suggested that PT during the initial days of VKA therapy is mainly indicative of the reduction of factor VII to its short half-life and the subsequent prolongation of PT occurring with the reduction of factors X and II. The PT monitoring of VKA treatment can be standardized by means of a calibration model that converts the PT ratio, measured with the local thromboplastin, into INR as described here:[3]

$$\text{INR} = (\text{Patient PT}/\text{Mean normal PT})^{\text{ISI}}$$

The International Sensitivity Index (ISI) corresponds to the degree of responsiveness of the given thromboplastin to vitamin K-dependent coagulation factors, compared to World Health Organization (WHO) international reference preparations.[3]

The starting dose of VKAs must be fixed after determining the baseline INR. During the initiation phase, it is recommended that INR be monitored every 2–4 days until the target range for therapeutic INR is noted for two consecutive values. Upon reaching stability, INR could be monitored weekly, and the interval could be increased to every 4 weeks upon the sustenance of INR stability in the therapeutic range.[2]

Maintenance of Therapeutic Anticoagulation—Time within Therapeutic Range

The maintenance of oral anticoagulation intensity within the target range is directly related to the desired benefits. The time within therapeutic range (TTR) is the best-recognized method for measuring the antithrombotic effectiveness of VKAs over time. The TTR is seen to be strongly associated with the primary clinical outcomes of hemorrhage or thrombosis, and an increase in TTR values has been associated with a reduction in the rates of myocardial infarction, stroke, and mortality. Hence, TTR can be considered a reliable measure of the high-quality maintenance of therapeutic anticoagulation.[4]

Routine monitoring helps in maintaining appropriate dosage of VKAs and in preventing over-coagulation and related adversities.[2]

Predictors of International Normalized Ratio Instability

Patient Characteristics

Variations in INR stability are largely influenced by patient-level factors as per data from large studies. Higher TTR attainment is associated with the use of advanced services at anticoagulation clinics, but studies indicate that approximately one-third of VKA patients have no accessibility to such services. Therefore, in clinical practice, knowledge of the predictors of INR instability is essential.[5]

Two of the most extensive studies that provided insight into factors influencing anticoagulation control include the SAMe-TT2R2 and the VARIA (Veterans AffaiRs study to Improve Anticoagulation) studies. The SAMe-

TT2R2 study conducted by Apostolaskis et al. used data on 1,061 AF patients from a previous trial to identify clinical factors associated with INR/TTR instability.[6] The VARIA study used data from over 124,000 veterans receiving warfarin, to evaluate the influence of patient characteristics on TTR. The factors associated with lower TTR in both the studies combined included:[7]

- Female gender
- Younger age
- Minority status
- Comorbid physical conditions
- Smoking
- Alcohol abuse
- Number of hospitalizations
- Comorbidities, such as heart failure, diabetes, chronic kidney disease, and chronic liver disease
- Treatment with β-blockers and verapamil.

Drugs

Vitamin K antagonists are known to be highly susceptible to drug-drug interactions. The concurrent use of certain medications could influence the effect of anticoagulation. For instance, drugs such as cholestyramine could reduce the absorption of warfarin, affecting its anticoagulant property. On the other hand, certain drugs are known to inhibit the clearance of the VKA, thereby potentiating the anticoagulant effect. Other drugs can increase the clearance of the VKA, thus inhibiting the anticoagulant effect.[3]

Vitamin K Intake

Changes in dietary vitamin K intake could impact the therapeutic stability of INR in patients on long-term VKA therapy. The intake of sufficient doses of vitamin K has been reported to be associated with increased INR stability.[3]

Challenges in Maintaining Target International Normalized Ratio

Genetics

Decreased enzymatic activity is associated with CYP2C9*2 and CYP2C9*3 polymorphisms in patients. This results in the slower metabolization of VKAs such as warfarin and, to a lesser degree, acenocoumarol; a 1.4- to 3.6-fold increased risk of supratherapeutic INR; and prolongation in the achievement of stable dosing.[5]

Adherence to Therapy

As per the American College of Chest Physicians (ACCP) guidelines, nonadherence to prescribed doses of medication is one of the most important variables in VKA INR stability. The individual risk factors of nonadherence include marital status, lack of transportation, employment status, mental health functioning, education level, poor cognitive functioning, and complexity of the drug regimen.[5]

MANAGING UNDER-COAGULATION OR OVER-COAGULATION WITH VKAS

Management of Under-Coagulation by Improving TTR

A number of initiatives for improving TTR could be taken; they are as follows:

- The general practitioner should be made aware of the problems faced by the patient that may hamper adequate and timely medication, such as poor cognitive function, comorbid conditions, and lack of social network. This facilitates the adoption of necessary adjustments to improve medication compliance[1]
- Accounting for comorbid conditions: In about 40% of anticoagulation cases, elderly people needed blood samples to be taken at home, owing to certain comorbid conditions; hence, there is a need for the involvement of nurses, family members, or neighbors, in the proper supervision of medicinal intake[1]
- Optimizing the INR test intervals and educating patients about the risks and benefits of the therapy can lead to adherence to several lifestyle recommendations and, subsequently, result in improved TTR.[8]

> Genetic polymorphisms and nonadherence to therapy are key factors responsible for INR instability.

MANAGEMENT OF OVERCOAGULATION-RELATED BLEEDING COMPLICATIONS

A major complication of overcoagulation is bleeding. International normalized ratio seems to be a major determinant of bleeding complications. It has also been reported that the bleeding risk increases with increase in INR; however, 50% of bleeding events occur at INR less than 4.0. According to observational studies, age-related comorbidities and a history of bleeding could also be related to the increased risk of bleeding. Table 1 provides guidelines for the management of VKA therapy during increased INR or bleeding complications.[9]

Table 1: Management guidelines for increased international normalized ratio (INR) in adult patients with or without bleeding[9]

Clinical setting	Action to be followed
When INR is higher than the therapeutic range but <5.0 and bleeding is absent	• Reduce the dose or omit the next dose of warfarin. When the INR approaches therapeutic range, resume therapy at a lower dose. • Dose reduction may not be necessary if the INR is only minimally above therapeutic range (up to 10%)
When INR is 5.0–9.0* and bleeding is absent	• Stop warfarin therapy; consider reasons for increased INR and patient-specific factors • Give vitamin K1 (1.0–2.0 mg orally or 0.5–1.0 mg intravenously) if bleeding risk is high • Take INR measurement within 24 hours;† once INR is in therapeutic range, resume warfarin at a reduced dose

Continued

Continued

Table 1: Management guidelines for increased international normalized ratio (INR) in adult patients with or without bleeding[9]

Clinical setting	Action to be followed
When INR is >9.0 and bleeding is absent	• Cease warfarin therapy where there is a low risk of bleeding; Administer orally 2.5–5.0 mg of vitamin K1 or intravenously 1.0 mg of vitamin K1. Measure INR in 6–12 hours, resume warfarin therapy at a reduced dose once INR <5.0 • Cease warfarin therapy where there is high risk of bleeding,[‡] give 1.0 mg vitamin K1 intravenously. Consider Prothrombinex-HT (25–50 IU/kg) and fresh frozen plasma (150–300 mL), measure INR in 6–12 h, resume warfarin therapy at a reduced dose once INR <5.0
Any clinically significant bleeding where warfarin induced coagulopathy is considered a contributing factor	• Stop warfarin therapy, give 5.0–10.0 mg vitamin K1 intravenously, as well as Prothrombinex-HT (25–50 IU/kg) and fresh frozen plasma (150–300 mL), continuously assess patient until INR <5.0, and bleeding stops[§] OR • Cease warfarin therapy if fresh frozen plasma is unavailable, give 5.0–10.0 mg vitamin K1 intravenously, and ProthrombinexHT (25–50 IU/kg), continuously assess patient until INR <5.0, and bleeding stops[§] OR • Cease warfarin therapy if Prothrombinex-HT is unavailable, give 5.0–10.0 mg vitamin K1 intravenously, and 10–15 mL/kg of fresh frozen plasma, continuously assess patient until INR <5.0, and bleeding stops[§]

*Bleeding risk increases exponentially from INR 5 to 9; INR ≥6 should be monitored closely.
†Vitamin K effect on INR can be expected within 6–12 hours.
‡Examples of patients in whom the bleeding risk would be expected to be high include those with active gastrointestinal disorders (such as peptic ulcer or inflammatory bowel disease), those receiving concomitant antiplatelet therapy, those who underwent a major surgical procedure within the preceding two weeks, and those with a low platelet count. See table 2 for list of bleeding risk factors.
§In all situations, carefully reassess the need for ongoing warfarin therapy.

Table 2: Risk factors for bleeding complications of anticoagulation therapy

Risk factor category	Specific risk factors
Age	>65 years
Cardiac	Uncontrolled hypertension
Gastrointestinal	History of gastrointestinal hemorrhage, active peptic ulcer, hepatic insufficiency
Hematologic/ oncologic	Thrombocytopenia (platelet count, $<50 \times 10^9$/L), platelet dysfunction, coagulation defect, underlying malignancy
Neurologic	History of stroke, cognitive, or psychological impairment

Continued

Continued

Table 2: Risk factors for bleeding complications of anticoagulation therapy

Risk factor category	Specific risk factors
Renal	Renal insufficiency
Trauma	Recent trauma, history of falls (>3 per within previous treatment year, or recurrent, injurious falls)
Alcohol	Excessive alcohol intake
Medications*	Aspirin, COX-I-specific nonsteroidal anti-inflammatory drugs (COX-II inhibitors do not impair platelet function, but can influence warfarin effect), "natural remedies" that interfere with hemostasis.

*Careful monitoring of warfarin effect is critical to minimise risk in patients taking multiple medications.

INITIATING ANTICOAGULANT THERAPY AFTER INTRACRANIAL HEMORRHAGE

Intracranial hemorrhage (ICH) is one of the most feared and life-threatening complications of OAC therapy. It remains uncertain as to how long the risk of ongoing bleeding persists after the initial onset of symptoms; therefore, the decision to resume anticoagulation therapy remains complicated. Recommendations by the European Stroke Initiative (ESI) and the American Heart Association (AHA) for anticoagulant therapy initiation post-ICH is indicated in table 3.[10]

Antidote to Vitamin K Antagonists

The incidence of severe bleeding in patients undergoing anticoagulant therapy or patients requiring emergency invasive procedures may need a reversal of anticoagulant treatment. The most straightforward approach to reversing the effect of conventional anticoagulants such as VKAs is the administration antidotes such as vitamin K or prothrombin complex concentrates. Vitamin K administration is crucial for the reversal of the anticoagulant effect in patients with clinically significant bleeding. Vitamin K can be given intravenously or orally, the former being more advantageous due to the rapid onset of treatment. The immediate correction of the INR is warranted during very serious or life-threatening bleeding. Vitamin K-dependent coagulation factors are administered in such situations. Prothrombin complex concentrates (PCCs) consisting entirely of vitamin K-dependent coagulation factors are particularly useful (Table 4).[11]

Table 3: American Heart Association and European Stroke Initiative recommendations for anticoagulant therapy initiation after intracranial hemorrhage[10]

The European Stroke Initiative	VKA therapy can be restarted after 10 to 14 days, depending on risk of thromboembolism and ICH recurrence in patients with a history of embolic stroke with AF
The American Heart Association	VKA can be restarted 7 to 10 days after ICH onset in patients with a very high risk of thromboembolism

VKA, vitamin K antagonist; ICH, intracranial hemorrhage; AF, atrial fibrillation.

Table 4: Agents used for reversal of vitamin K antagonist therapy[11]

	Time until restoration of hemostasis after cessation of therapeutic dose	Reversing agent	Remark
Vitamin K antagonists	• Warfarin: 60–80 h • Acenocoumarol: 18–24 h • Phenprocoumon: 8–10 days	• Vitamin K intravenously; reversal in 12–16 h • Vitamin K orally; reversal in 24 h • PCCs; immediate reversal	• Dose of vitamin K or PCCs depend on INR and bodyweight

PCCs, prothrombin complex concentrates; INR, international normalized ratio.

THE AMERICAN COLLEGE OF CHEST PHYSICIANS EVIDENCE-BASED CLINICAL PRACTICE GUIDELINES FOR MANAGEMENT OF INR FLUCTUATIONS

The most important objective after OAC therapy initiation is the achievement (and maintenance) of a therapeutic INR, and the improvement of the percent of time spent in the therapeutic range (TTR). The narrow therapeutic window of VKAs and their susceptibility to food, drugs, alcohol, and other patient-related factors makes high-quality anticoagulation therapy management a necessity.[8] Table 5 provides evidence-based guidelines for the effective maintenance of therapeutic INR as recommended by the ACCP.[12]

Table 5: The American College of Chest Physicians guidelines for maintaining therapeutic international normalized ratio[12]

Patient type	Recommendation
Those initiating VKA therapy	Avoid routine use of pharmacogenetic testing for guiding VKA doses
Those with consistently stable INR during VKA therapy	INR testing frequency of up to 12 weeks instead of every 4 weeks
Those on VKA therapy and presenting a single out-of-range INR of <0.5 below or above therapeutic range	Continuation of present dosage with INR testing within 1–2 weeks
Those with stable therapeutic INR and a single subtherapeutic INR	Avoid routine bridging with heparin
Those taking VKAs	Avoid routine intake of vitamin K supplementation
Those who are motivated and competent in self-management strategies	Use patient self-monitoring system rather than outpatient INR monitoring
Those on maintenance VKA therapy	Dosing decisions to be made using validated decision tools

Continued

Continued

Table 5: The American College of Chest Physicians guidelines for maintaining therapeutic international normalized ratio[12]

Patient type	Recommendation
Those on VKA therapy	• Avoid concurrent medication, such as non-steroidal antiinflammatory drugs, antiplatelet agents, and certain antibiotics • Maintain optimal therapeutic INR range of 2.0 to 3.0 (target INR: 2.5) rather than a lower (INR<2) or higher (INR 3.0–5.0) range

INR, international normalized ratio; VKA, vitamin K antagonist.

KEY POINTS

- Monitoring anticoagulant efficacy is essential for fixing the initial dose of VKA therapy and subsequent maintenance doses, for optimal benefit without complications
- The TTR is the most widely used criterion for measuring the quality of therapeutic anticoagulation
- Various intra- and interpatient-related factors influence INR stability and pose a challenge in maintaining the target INR
- High-quality anticoagulation management through evidence-based guidelines ensures the therapeutic safety and efficacy of VKAs.

REFERENCES

1. Ten Cate H. Monitoring new oral anticoagulants, managing thrombosis, or both? Thromb Haemost. 2012;107(5):803-5.
2. Monitoring oral anticoagulation therapy. J Assoc Physicians India. 2014;62(6 Suppl):30-3.
3. Ageno W, Gallus AS, Wittkowsky A, et al. Oral anticoagulant therapy: Antithrombotic Therapy and Prevention of Thrombosis, 9th ed: American College of Chest Physicians Evidence-Based Clinical Practice Guidelines. Chest. 2012;141(2):e44S-88S
4. Phillips K, Ansell J. Outpatient management of oral vitamin K antagonist therapy: Defining and measuring high-quality management. Expert Rev Cardiovasc Ther. 2008;6(1):57-70.
5. Schein JR, White CM, Nelson WW, et al. Vitamin K antagonist use: evidence of the difficulty of achieving and maintaining target INR range and subsequent consequences. Thromb J. 2016;14:14.
6. Apostolakis S, Sullivan RM, Olshansky B, et al. Factors affecting quality of anticoagulation control among patients with atrial fibrillation on warfarin: the SAMe-TT_2R_2 score. Chest. 2013;144(5):1555-63.
7. Rose AJ, Hylek EM, Ozonoff A, et al. Patient characteristics associated with oral anticoagulation control: results of the Veterans AffaiRs Study to Improve Anticoagulation (VARIA). J Thromb Haemost. 2010;8(10):2182-91.
8. Smith DE, Lip GY, Lane DA. Strategies to improve oral anticoagulation management. Chest. 2011;140(2):281-2.
9. Baker RI, Coughlin PB, Gallus AS, et al. Warfarin reversal: consensus guidelines, on behalf of the Australasian Society of Thrombosis and Haemostasis. Med J Aust. 2004;181(9):492-7.
10. Goldstein JN, Greenberg SM. Should anticoagulation be resumed after intracerebral hemorrhage? Cleve Clin J Med. 2010;77(11):791-9.
11. Levi M, Eerenberg E, Kamphuisen P. Bleeding risk and reversal strategies for old and new anticoagulants and antiplatelet agents. J Thromb Haemost. 2011;9(9):1705-12.
12. Holbrook A, Schulman S, Witt DM, et al. Evidence-based management of anticoagulant therapy: Antithrombotic Therapy and Prevention of Thrombosis, 9th ed: American College of Chest Physicians Evidence-Based Clinical Practice Guidelines. Chest. 2012;141(2 Suppl):52-84.

7

Initiation and Maintenance of Vitamin K Antagonist Therapy

Nirmal Kumar

INTRODUCTION

Vitamin K antagonists (VKAs), such as acenocoumarol, have a wide range of indications for prophylaxis and treatment of thromboembolic diseases. High-quality dosing management of coumarin anticoagulants (COAs) is essential during long-term therapy. However, a narrow therapeutic range and significant inter- and intra-patient variability, along with inter-ethnic differences in stabilizing doses, pose a huge challenge in maintaining the optimal dosing of COAs. Routine monitoring of prothrombin time (PT) and international normalized ratio (INR) measurements are required, as lower doses may lead to undercoagulation and decreased efficacy, while overdosing may lead to increased risk of bleeding incidences. The risk of complications due to under dosing and overdosing is particularly high during the initial phase of COA therapy. Therefore, it is important to predict the correct initial loading dose and subsequent stabilizing doses of COA to avail optimal therapy benefits devoid of adverse events.[1] This chapter deals with different aspects of appropriate dosing and the administration of COAs such as acenocoumarol.

DOSING AND ADMINISTRATION OF ACENOCOUMAROL

Acenocoumarol is usually administered as a once-daily oral dose at a specific time each day, usually in the evening, and there is a gap of 2 hours between the drug dose and the last meal. Monitoring dosage requirement is essential due to the differential sensitivity and significant variability of the anticoagulant effect among patients. Acenocoumarol should not be administered in cases where there is an unavailability of resources for regular monitoring of PT/INR for dosage adjustments.[2]

Baseline Testing[3]

Prior to initiation of acenocoumarol, patients should have appropriate baseline testing, which includes:

- Prothrombin time with an INR and activated partial thromboplastin time (aPTT), to obtain a baseline value for monitoring, and to identify any underlying abnormalities
- Complete blood count, including platelet count, to obtain a baseline and identify thrombocytopenia

- Serum creatinine, to estimate the glomerular filtration rate (GFR)
- Liver function tests, to identify potential alterations in warfarin metabolism (or hemostasis)
- A urine (or serum) pregnancy test for women of childbearing potential, because of the risk of teratogenicity.

Initial Dosing[3,4]

Expert Opinion

In Western literature, the recommended initial dose of VKA is 4 mg and goes up to 8 mg per day, but in the Indian scenario patients are unable to tolerate such a high dose. Clinical practice dosages in India usually start with smaller doses to begin with, and are titrated according to PT/INR.
For patients starting acenocoumarol therapy, an initial daily dose of 2 mg, rather than higher doses or "loading" doses is recommended, unless the patient is known from previous experience to require higher doses.

The rationale for the avoidance of higher initial doses is that higher doses generally do not result in more rapid therapeutic anticoagulation or improved outcomes, but these higher doses were more likely to lead to a supratherapeutic INR, which can increase the risk of bleeding. Additionally, there is a theoretical concern that higher initial doses might cause more dramatic reductions in the anticoagulant factors protein S and protein C, leading to a greater transient procoagulant state.
The initial dose is further individualized to take into account factors that may lead to excessive anticoagulation or increased risk of bleeding such as older age, variability in metabolism, and vitamin K dietary status. Some specific recommendations are as follows:

- For an otherwise healthy adult, the typical dosage consists of 2 mg daily on days 1 and 2
- For an adult who is frail, elderly (e.g., woman >70 years, man >80 years), malnourished, has liver or kidney disease or heart failure, or is receiving a medication known to increase VKA sensitivity such as amiodarone, a lower dosage is recommended
- A higher initial dose may be required in some individuals such as those previously receiving VKA anticoagulation and requiring a higher-than-average dose.

Protocol for Dose Titration of Acenocoumarol

Therapeutic INR can be easily maintained with a single daily dose of acenocoumarol. Table 1 provides the protocol for the maintenance of the therapeutic INR with a single daily dose of acenocoumarol, through appropriate dose titrations.[5]

Maintenance Dosage

Maintenance therapy dosage requirements must be based on regular laboratory estimations, due to significant inter-patient variability in blood

Table 1: Dose titration protocol of acenocoumarol[5]

International normalized ratio	To current dose of acenocoumarol; INR monitoring
<1.3	Add 1 mg/day; Repeat INR post 1 week
1.4–2	Add 0/5 mg/day; Repeat INR post 1 week
2.1–3	Continue with cut-tent dose
3.1–3.5	Decrease by 0.5 mg/day; Repeat INR post 1 week
3.6–4	Decrease by 1 mg/day; Repeat INR post 1 week
> 4	Stop therapy for 3 days; Repeat INR
If INR remains >4	Withhold therapy till the desirable INR range is achieved
If INR <4 on repeated measurement	Follow as above

INR, international normalized ratio.

Table 2: Recommended INR for oral anticoagulation therapy in patients with different indications[2]

Recommended international normalized ratio	2.0–3.0	2.0–3.5
Indication	• Prophylaxis and treatment of venous thromboembolism (including pulmonary embolism) • Atrial fibrillation • Postmyocardial infarction (with increased risk for thromboembolic complications) • Bioprosthetic heart valves • Secondary prophylaxis in patients with antiphospholipid syndrome	• Antiphospholipid syndrome patients with venous thromboembolism on therapeutic vitamin K antagonist • Mechanical heart valves

INR, international normalized ratio.

coagulation time. Dosage adjustments must be carried out based on the Quick value of INR at routine intervals, in order to maintain the target INR in the therapeutic range. The maintenance dosage usually ranges between 1 mg and 8 mg, depending on the individual patient's condition (Table 2).[2]

Conversion from Heparin Therapy

Initial treatment with heparin is recommended in clinical situations that require immediate anticoagulation. This is due to the delayed anticoagulation effect of acenocoumarol. Conversion to acenocoumarol may begin concurrently with heparin therapy or may require delayed initiation, depending on the clinical situation. Full-dose heparin therapy is prescribed along with acenocoumarol initiation for at least 4 days in order to maintain continuous anticoagulation. Concomitant treatment with heparin is continued until INR stability in the target range has been achieved for at least two consecutive days. This transition phase requires close monitoring of anticoagulation.[2]

Conversion to acenocoumarol may begin concurrently with heparin therapy, or may require delayed initiation.[2]

Genetic Polymorphisms and Their Impact on Acenocoumarol Dosage[1]

The role of genetics is substantial in drug dosage variability; genetics plays a key role in the achievement of the therapeutic INR range. It has been reported that over 30 genes are actively involved in the drug metabolism of COAs. The most important are the genes encoding the cytochrome P450 drug-metabolizing enzyme–CYP2C9 and the gene encoding the drug target enzyme–VKORC1. Single nucleotide polymorphisms (SNPs) in VKORC1 account for 30% of the drug dosage variance, while two nonsynonymous SNPs (*2,*3) in the CYP2C9 region account for 12% of the drug variance, according to previous studies. However, complex sets of both environmental and genetic determinants influence the individual therapeutic drug dosage. Therefore, a pharmacogenetic dosing algorithm using multiple and linear stepwise regression analyses has been proposed, based on genetic as well as clinical factors, for a more accurate prediction of acenocoumarol dosage (Table 3).[1]

Table 3: Pharmacogenetic dosing algorithm for therapeutic dosing of acenocoumarol[1]

Method	Model, x variables	Regression equation	p value	R^2 for model (%)
Multiple regression	VKORC1, CYP4F2, CYP2C9*2, CYP2C9*3, GGCX genotypes, weight, height, sex, age, body surface area, smoking status and indication for surgery	Dose (mg/day) = 3.082–0.013 (smoking status, 1 for smoker and 0 for nonsmoker) -0.433 (sex, 1 for male and 0 for female) -0.004 (age) + indication (0.327 for DVR and -0.092 for AVR) +0.026 (height) +0.151 (weight) -7.660 (body surface area) -0.862 (VKORC1 GA) -2.257 (VKORC1 AA) -0.049 (CYP2C9*2 CT) -0.456 (CYP2C9*3 AC) +0.449 (CYP4F2 GA) +0.230 (CYP4F2 AA) +0.245 (GGCX CG) +1.055 (GGCX GG)	<0.001	41.4

Continued

Continued

Table 3: Pharmacogenetic dosing algorithm for therapeutic dosing of acenocoumarol[1]

Method	Model, x variables	Regression equation	p value	R^2 for model (%)
Linear stepwise regression	Weight, sex	Dose (mg/day) = 1.418 + 0.038 (weight)-0.564 (1 for male, 0 for female)	<0.001	12.5
Linear stepwise regression	VKORC1 genotype, weight	Dose (mg/day) = 0.755 + 0.896 (VKORC1 GG) - 1.396 (VKORC1 AA) + 0.033 (weight)	<0.001	31.0
Linear stepwise regression	VKORC1 genotype, weight, sex	Dose (mg/day) = 0.192 + 0.879 (VKORC1 GG) - 1.443 (VKORC1 AA) ± 0.04 (weight) + 0.569 (1 for male, 0 for female)	<0.001	34.9
Linear stepwise regression	VKORC1, CYP4F2 genotypes weight, sex	Dose (mg/day) = 2.329 (VKORC1 GG) +1.45 (VKORC1 GA) +0.362 (CYP4F2 GA) +0.038 (weight) -0.535 (1 for male, 0 for female) -0.799	<0.001	37.0

The 2012 American College of Chest Physicians (ACCP) guidelines, however, do not recommend routine use of genotyping for guiding the dosing of VKAs.[3]

Missed Dose[2]

Acenocoumarol's anticoagulant effects seem to persist beyond 24 hours. In case of a missed dose, the patients are to be advised to take the prescribed dose of missed medication as soon as possible on the same day. Doubling the prescribed daily dose in order to make up for the missed dose is not advisable, and any further action in this regard needs to be approved by the patient's physician.

> A missed dose must be taken as soon as possible on the same day.[2]

Treatment Discontinuation[2]

The risk of reactive hypercoagulability is minimal after acenocoumarol withdrawal; therefore, abrupt withdrawal can be undertaken instead of a gradual tapering down of dosage. However, certain high-risk populations (postmyocardial infarction) and other extremely rare cases may require the gradual withdrawal of dosage, due to a higher possibility of "rebound" hypercoagulability.

> Abrupt discontinuation of treatment can be done instead of giving gradual diminishing doses.[2]

DOSING IN SPECIAL POPULATIONS[2]

Patients with specific comorbid conditions may require special precautions with respect to acenocoumarol administration. Table 4 provides specific acenocoumarol dosing recommendations for some special populations.

Table 6: Acenocoumarol dosage for special indications[2]

Indication	Recommendation
Renal impairment	• Not recommended in cases of severe renal impairment due to heightened risk of bleeding • Use in patients with mild-to-moderate renal impairment advised with caution
Hepatic impairment	• Not recommended in cases of severe hepatic impairment due to heightened risk of bleeding • Use in patients with mild-to-moderate hepatic impairment advised with caution
Heart failure	• Caution in exercising dosage in cases of severe heart failure is recommended, as hepatic congestion may lead to a reduction in the activation of gamma-carboxylation of coagulation factors • Increased dosage may be required upon reversal of hepatic congestion
Hematological	• Caution must be exercised in dosage recommendation for patients with known or suspected protein C or protein S deficiency
Conditions such as thyrotoxicosis, tumors, renal disease, infections, and inflammation	• Strict medical supervision recommended due to reduction in protein binding of acenocoumarol

OTHER INDICATIONS AND RECOMMENDATIONS

- Subcutaneous and intravenous injections are preferable to subcutaneous injections during anticoagulant treatment, to reduce the risk of hematomas
- Caution in dosing must be followed during diagnostic or therapeutic procedures that may require the shortening of PT/INR such as angiography, lumbar puncture, and minor surgery or tooth extractions
- Elderly patients may require lower initial and maintenance doses. Elderly patients on anticoagulant therapy should be monitored with special care.

KEY POINTS

- It is important to predict the correct initial dose and subsequent maintenance dosage of anticoagulant treatment, to avail maximum therapy benefits without complications
- Acenocoumarol treatment should be carried out with routine INR/PT monitoring
- A variety of environmental and genetic factors may influence individual dosing requirements
- Special populations with specific conditions may require specialized dosing recommendations.

REFERENCES

1. Rathore SS, Agarwal SK, Pande S, Singh SK, Mittal T, Mittall B. Therapeutic dosing of acenocoumarol: Proposal of a population specific pharmacogenetic dosing algorithm and its validation in North Indians. PLoS One. 2012;7(5):e37844.
2. Trailokya A. Acenocoumarol in thromoembolic disorders. Cardiovasc Pharm Open Access. 2015;4:157.
3. Maddali S, Biring T, Bluhm J, Kopecky S, Krueger K, Larson T, et al. Antithrombotic therapy supplement. ICSI. 2013:88.
4. Hoffman R, Benz EJ, Shattil SJ, Furie B, Silberstein LE, McGlave P, et al. Hematology: Basic Principles and Practice, 3rd edition. New York: Churchill Livingstone; 2000. p. 2040.
5. Anticoagulant agents. J Assoc Physicians India. 2014;62:10-8.

8

Anticoagulation in Nonvalvular Atrial Fibrillation

Ummer K

INTRODUCTION

Atrial fibrillation (AF) is one of the most clinically noted forms of cardiac arrhythmia affecting 1–2% of the global population; the prevalence of AF is estimated to double in the next 50 years, with the increase in the aging population. A fivefold increase in ischemic stroke has been associated with AF, with one in five of all strokes linked to this arrhythmia.[1] This chapter focuses on the clinical evidence supporting the therapeutic use of oral vitamin K antagonists (VKAs) in the prevention of stroke, as well as published guidelines aimed at the effective management of nonvalvular AF and the prevention of thromboembolism in patients with AF.

RISK OF STROKE IN ATRIAL FIBRILLATION: CLINICAL EVIDENCE

The role of AF as a powerful independent risk factor for ischemic stroke was investigated in the Framingham study, which assessed the influence of nonrheumatic AF, hypertension, coronary heart disease, and cardiac failure on stroke incidence in 5,070 participants after 34 years of follow-up. The age-adjusted incidence of stroke was compared to subjects who were free from any cardiovascular conditions. Atrial fibrillation was associated with a fivefold excess stroke incidence, higher than any other risk factor assessed (Fig. 1). This impact of AF was also found to be independent of other cardiovascular abnormalities, and its influence seems to increase with age, contrary to other cardiovascular comorbidities.[2]

PREDICTION OF RISK OF STROKE IN ATRIAL FIBRILLATION

$CHADS_2$ Score

An increased risk of stroke is associated with patients with AF; however, age and comorbid conditions may influence the absolute rate of stroke. The Atrial Fibrillation Investigators (AFI) formed a unified stroke classification scheme known as the $CHADS_2$ score by combining risk factors from prior studies and then testing their validity in a cohort of 1,773 Medicare-aged patients, over 2,121 patient years.[3] The $CHADS_2$ risk index uses a point-based system of risk assessment (Table 1). The adjusted annual stroke risk rate corresponding to the $CHADS_2$ score is depicted in figure 2, assuming that no aspirin was taken during the course of the study.[1]

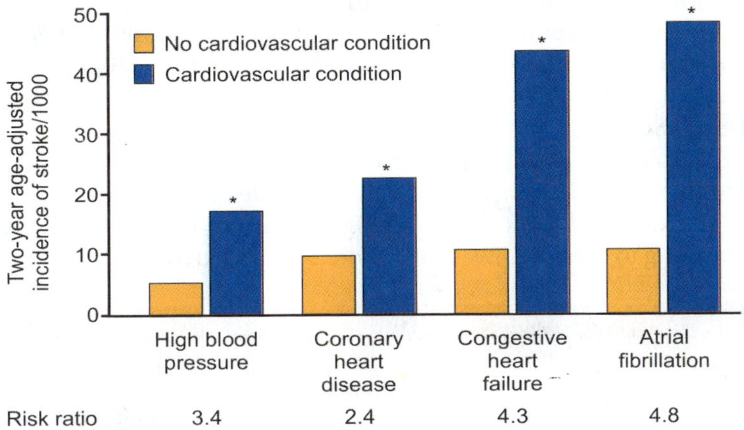

*p <0.001 different from unity.[2]

Fig. 1: Two-year age-adjusted incidence of stroke according to the presence or absence of cardiovascular condition.

Table 1: $CHADS_2$ score: Stroke risk assessment in atrial fibrillation[1]	
Score	**$CHADS_2$ risk criteria**
1 point	Congestive heart failure
1 point	Hypertension
1 point	Age >75
1 point	Diabetes mellitus
2 points	Stroke/transient ischemic attack

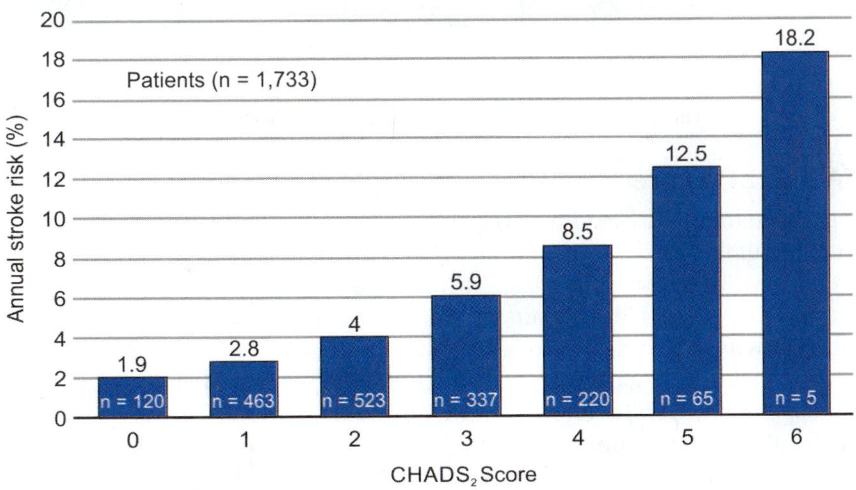

Fig. 2: $CHADS_2$ score and corresponding annual stroke risk

CHA_2DS_2-VASc score

A more recent strategy for the risk factor-based stratification of patients with non-valvular AF includes "major (definitive)" risk factors [such as prior stroke, transient ischemic attack (TIA), and age ≥75 years] and "clinically relevant nonmajor" risk factors (such as female gender, age 65–75 years, and atherosclerotic vascular disease). This approach is known by the acronym CHA_2DS_2-VASc [congestive heart failure, hypertension, age ≥75 (doubled), diabetes, stroke (doubled), vascular disease, and age 65–74 years, and sex category (female)]. The CHA_2DS_2-VASc risk index also uses a point-based system of risk assessment (Table 2). The adjusted annual stroke risk rate corresponding to the CHA_2DS_2-VASc score is depicted in figure 3.[1]

Table 2: CHA_2DS_2-VASc score: stroke risk assessment in atrial fibrillation[1]

Score	1 point	2 point
CHA_2DS_2-VASc risk criteria	• Congestive heart failure • Hypertension • Age ≥75 • Diabetes mellitus • Stroke/transient ischemic attack • Vascular disease	• Age ≥75 • Stroke/transient ischemic attack

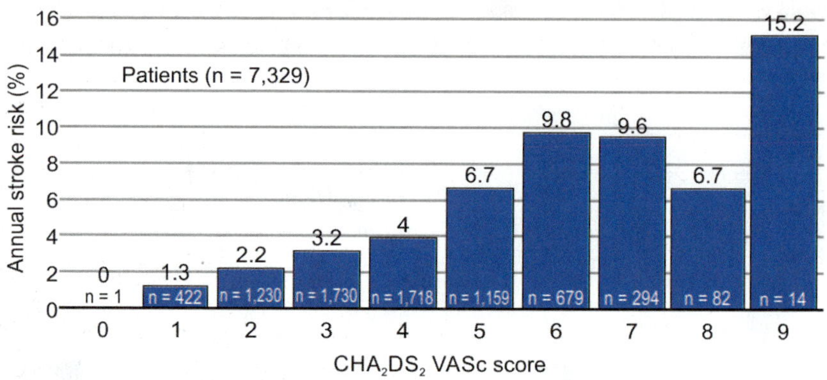

Fig. 3: CHA_2DS_2-VASc score and corresponding annual stroke risk

HAS-BLED Score

The assessment of bleeding risk should be considered a prerequisite for anticoagulant therapy initiation. The EuroHeart Survey estimated the 1-year risk of major bleeding (intracranial, hospitalization, hemoglobin decrease >2 /L, and/or transfusion) in a real-world cohort of 3,978 European subjects with AF and developed a bleeding risk score termed HAS-BLED [Hypertension, Abnormal renal/liver function, Stroke, Bleeding history or predisposition, Labile international normalized ratio, Elderly (65 years), Drugs/alcohol concomitantly] (Table 3). This practical tool may be used for assessing the individualized bleeding risk among AF patients and aid in arriving at clinical decisions regarding antithrombotic therapy.[1]

Table 3: HAS-BLED bleeding risk score[1]		
Letter	Clinical characteristic	Points awarded
H	Hypertension	1
A	Abnormal renal or liver function (1 point each)	1 or 2
S	Stroke	1
B	Bleeding	1
L	Labile international normalized ratios	1
E	Elderly (e.g., age >65 years)	1
D	Drugs or alcohol (1 point each)	1 or 2

ANTICOAGULATION FOR STROKE PREVENTION IN ATRIAL FIBRILLATION: CLINICAL EVIDENCE

Chronic oral anticoagulant treatment, which aims at suppression of the coagulation cascade and platelet activation, is a highly credible prophylactic measure for the management of AF in patients who are at high risk for thromboembolic events.[4]

Five large randomized trials published between the late 1980s and through the 1990s evaluated the efficacy of oral VKAs, mainly for the primary prevention of thromboembolism in patients with nonvalvular AF. A 6th trial, the European Atrial Fibrillation Trial (EAFT), investigated secondary prevention among patients with recent nondisabling stroke or TIA. Patients with persistent, permanent, paroxysmal, or intermittent AF were included in these studies. Patients with valvular AF were excluded. A relative risk reduction ranging from 52% to 82% was observed in the primary prevention trials, and a relative risk reduction of 66% was observed in EAFT (secondary prevention trial). Table 4 summarizes the results of all the six studies.[5]

Table 4: Anticoagulation therapy vs. control for stroke prevention in atrial fibrillation: Summary of results from 6 randomized trials[5]

Trials	**Annual stroke rate (%)**			
	INR target	**Control**	**Warfarin**	**Relative risk reduction**
Atrial Fibrillation, Aspirin, and Anticoagulation (AFASAK) trial	2.8–4.2	5.5	1.6	71*
Boston Area Anticoagulation Trial for Atrial Fibrillation (BAATAF)	2.0–3.0	3.0	0.4	86*
Stroke Prevention in Atrial Fibrillation (SPAF-I)	2.0–4.5	7.4	2.3	69*
Canadian Atrial Fibrillation Anticoagulation (CAFA)	2.0–3.0	5.2	2.5	52
Stroke Prevention in Nonrheumatic Atrial Fibrillation (SPINAF)	2.0–3.0	4.3	0.9	79*
European Atrial Fibrillation Trial (EAFT)	2.5–4.0	12.3	3.9	66*

*p <0.05

ANTIPLATELETS VERSUS ANTICOAGULANTS FOR STROKE PREVENTION IN ATRIAL FIBRILLATION: CLINICAL EVIDENCE

Oral anticoagulants and antiplatelet agents have proven efficacy with respect to secondary stroke prevention in patients at high risk for vascular events. However, the suspected cardioembolic mechanism of AF-related strokes warrants special consideration during primary stroke prevention in patients with nonvalvular AF.[6]

A meta-analysis that included eight randomized trials (n = 9,598) investigated the long-term efficacy of oral anticoagulant therapy compared to antiplatelet treatment in patients with non-valvular AF with no prior history of stroke or TIA. The mean overall follow-up was 1.9 years/participant. An overall lower risk of all stroke [odds ratio (OR) 0.68, 95% confidence interval (CI) 0.54–0.85), ischemic stroke (OR 0.53, 95% CI 0.41–0.68), and systemic emboli (OR 0.48, 95% CI 0.25–0.90) was noted with oral anticoagulant treatment compared to antiplatelet therapy.

VITAMIN K ANTAGONISTS IN STROKE PREVENTION: TRANSLATING CLINICAL TRIALS INTO PRACTICE

The efficacy of oral VKAs over aspirin or placebo in stroke prevention has been suggested in various randomized trials. However, there exist concerns among clinicians over the efficacy of anticoagulation therapy in actual clinical practice, where less intensive anticoagulation monitoring may be undertaken in sick patients. Several observational studies have been conducted in order to test the safety and efficacy of antithrombotic therapy in preventing thromboembolism in AF and to determine whether the results from randomized trials could be duplicated in clinical practice.[5]

In a 2-year prospective cohort study, 167 patients with AF and at high risk of stroke receiving anticoagulation treatment in clinical practice were compared with patients from five randomized controlled trials. The results indicated that the incidence of stroke in patients receiving warfarin in the study group (2.0% per year, 0.7–4.4%) was comparable to that observed in pooled studies (1.4%, 0.8–2.3%). The rate of major hemorrhage was also found to be similar.[7]

Two studies conducted in a hospital setting found warfarin to be significantly more effective compared to aspirin or no antithrombotic therapy for secondary stroke prevention, in high-risk patients with AF. Table 5 provides the results of these two observational studies.[8,9]

The Anticoagulation and Risk Factors in Atrial Fibrillation (ATRIA) study, a contemporary population-based cohort of 13,559 ambulatory adults, diagnosed with nonvalvular AF in northern California, collected longitudinal information on warfarin use along with associated clinical outcomes. Of these 13,559 patients, 11,526 were evaluated for the effect of warfarin on the risk of thromboembolism, hemorrhage, and death within a clinical setting. The study

Table 5: Summary of results from two observational studies evaluating the efficacy of anticoagulant treatment in the clinical setting[8-9]

Study	Setting	Population	Ischemic stroke					
			N	Warfarin risk (%) (95% CI)	N	Aspirin risk (%) (95% CI)	N	No risk (%) (95% CI)
Evans, 2001	Hospital	386 acute stroke patients with AF (214 warfarin, 172 aspirin)	19	4.2 (2.3–6.2)*†	33	9.2 (6.1–12.4)*	–	N/A
Evans, 2000	Hospital	288 ischemic stroke patients with AF eligible for and given warfarin	16	3.8 (2.0–5.6)*† (on warfarin)	–	N/A	16	8.5 (4.3–12.7)† (off warfarin)

*Target international normalized ratio of 2.0 to 3.0.
†Annual event rate.

found warfarin therapy to be associated with a 51% (95% CI, 39–60%) lower risk of thromboembolism compared to no anticoagulant or aspirin therapy. The study concluded that results from randomized trials could be translated effectively in clinical settings, for patients with AF.[10]

CURRENT RECOMMENDATION FOR ANTICOAGULANT THERAPY

As per the European Society of Cardiologists (ESC), the presence or absence of risk factors must be the basis of antithrombotic therapy recommendations. The initial risk assessment should be carried out by means of a $CHADS_2$ stroke risk stratification scheme. Dose-adjusted VKA therapy is recommended in patients with a $CHADS_2$ score of more than or equal to 2, in order to achieve an international normalized ratio target range of 2.0–3.0, unless contraindicated. A more comprehensive risk-based strategy such as CHA_2DS_2-VASc is recommended in patients with a $CHADS_2$ score of 0–1 (Table 6 and Flowchart 1).[1]

GUIDELINES AND RECOMMENDATIONS

The recommendations for prevention of thromboembolism by the ESC and the summary of recommendations for risk-based antithrombotic therapy as per the American College of Cardiology (ACC)/American Heart Association (AHA)/Heart Rhythm Society (HRS) 2014 guidelines have been outlined in tables 7 and 8, respectively.[11,12]

Table 6: Thromboprophylaxis recommendations in patients with atrial fbrillation[1]

Risk category	No risk factors	One clinically relevant nonmajor risk factor	One major risk factor or ≥2 clinically relevant nonmajo
CHA_2DS_2-VASc score	0	1	≥2
Recommended antithrombotic therapy	Either aspirin 75–325 mg daily or no antithrombotic therapy. Preferred: No antithrombotic therapy rather than aspirin	Either Oral anticoagulant or aspirin 75–325 mg daily. Preferred: Oral anticoagulant rather than aspirin	Oral anticoagulant

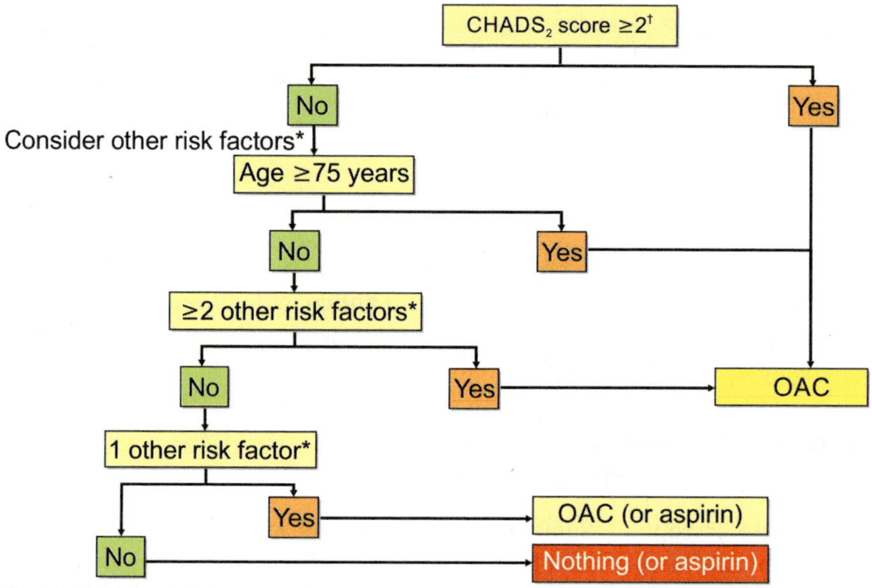

OAC, Oral anticoagulant.

†Congestive heart failure, hypertension; age >75 years diabetes; stroke/transient ischemic attack thromboembolism (doubled).

*Other clinically relevant nonmajor risk factors: Age 65–74, female sex, vascular disease.

Flowchart 1: Oral anticoagulant use in patients with atrial fibrillation[1]

Table 7: European Society of Cardiology recommendations for prevention of thromboembolism[11]

Recommendations	Class	Level
Recommendations for prevention of thromboembolism in nonvalvular AF—general		
Antithrombotic therapy to prevent thromboembolism is recommended for all patients with AF, except in those patients (both male and female) who are at low risk (aged <65 years and lone AF), or with contraindications	I	A

Continued

Continued

Table 7: European Society of Cardiology recommendations for prevention of thromboembolism[11]

Recommendations	Class	Level
The choice of antithrombotic therapy should be based upon the absolute risks of stroke/thromboembolism and bleeding and the net clinical benefit for a given patient	I	A
The CHA_2DS_2-VASc score is recommended as a means of assessing stroke risk in nonvalvular AF	I	A
In patients with a CHA_2DS_2-VASc score of 0 (i.e., aged <65 years with lone AF) who are at low risk, with none of the risk factors, no antithrombotic therapy is recommended	I	B
In patients with a CHA_2DS_2-VASc score ≥2, OAC therapy withone of the following is recommended, unless contraindicated: • Adjusted-dose VKA (INR 2–3) • A direct thrombin inhibitor (dabigatran) • An oral factor Xa inhibitor (e.g., rivaroxaban, apixaban)	I	A
In patients with a CHA_2DS_2-VASc score of 1, OAC therapy with one of the following should be considered, based upon an assessment of the risk of bleeding complications and patient preferences: • Adjusted-dose VKA (INR 2–3) • A direct thrombin inhibitor (dabigatran) • An oral factor Xa inhibitor (e.g., rivaroxaban, apixaban)	IIa	A
Female patients who are aged <65 and have lone AF (but still have a CHA_2DS_2-VASc score of 1 by virtue of their gender) are low risk and no antithrombotic therapy should be considered	IIa	B
When patients refuse the use of any OAC (whether VKAs or NOACs), antiplatelet therapy should be considered, using combination therapy with aspirin 75–100 mg plus clopidogrel 75 mg daily (where there is a low risk of bleeding) or—less effectively—aspirin 75–325 mg daily	IIa	B
Assessment of the risk of bleeding is recommended when prescribing antithrombotic therapy (whether with VKA, NOAC, aspirin/clopidogrel, or aspirin)	I	A
The HAS-BLED score should be considered as a calculation to assess bleeding risk, whereby a score ≥3 indicates "high risk" and some caution and regular review is needed, following the initiation of antithrombotic therapy, whether with OAC or antiplatelet therapy (LoE = A)	IIa	A B
Correctable risk factors for bleeding [e.g., uncontrolled blood pressure, labile INRs if the patient was on a VKA, concomitant drugs (aspirin, NSAIDs, etc.), alcohol, etc.] should be addressed (LoE = B)		
Use of the HAS-BLED score should be used to identify modifiable bleeding risks that need to be addressed, but should not be used on its own to exclude patients from OAC therapy (LoE = B)		

Continued

Continued

Table 7: European Society of Cardiology recommendations for prevention of thromboembolism[11]

Recommendations	Class	Level
The risk of major bleeding with antiplatelet therapy (with aspirin-clopidogrel combination therapy and—especially in the elderly—also with aspirin monotherapy) should be considered as being similar to OAC	IIa	B
Recommendations for prevention of thromboembolism in nonvalvular AF—pericardioversion		
For patients with AF of ≥48 h duration, or when the duration of AF is unknown, OAC therapy (e.g., VKA with INR 2–3 or dabigatran) is recommended for ≥3 weeks prior to and for ≥4 weeks after cardioversion, regardless of the method (electrical or oral/intravenous pharmacological)	I	B
In patients with risk factors for stroke or AF recurrence, OAC therapy, whether with dose-adjusted VKA (INR 2–3) or a NOAC, should be continued lifelong irrespective of the apparent maintenance of sinus rhythm following cardioversion	I	B

AF, atrial fibrillation; OAC, oral anticoagulant; INR, international normalized ratio; NOAC, novel oral anticoagulants; VKA, vitamin K antagonist; LoE, level of evidence.

Class I: Evidence that given treatment is useful, effective.
Class II: Conflicting evidence about usefulness/effectiveness of given treatment.
Class IIa: Weight of evidence in favour of usefulness/efficacy.
Class IIb: Usefullness/effectiveness less well established by evidence.
Class III: Evidence that given treatment is not useful/effective, may be harmful in some cases.
Level A: Data derived from multiple randomized clinical trails or meta-analysis.
Level B: Data derived from single randomized clinical trial or large nonrandomized studies.
Level C: Consensus of opinion of experts and/or small studies, retrospective studies, and registries.

Table 8: The 2014 American Heart Association/American College of Cardiology/Heart Rhythm Society guidelines for risk-based antithrombotic treatment[12]

Recommendations	CoR	LoE
Antithrombotic therapy based on shared decision making, discussion of risks of stroke and bleeding, and patient's preferences	I	C
Selection of antithrombotic therapy based on risk of thromboembolism	I	B
CHA_2DS_2-VASc score recommended to assess stroke risk	I	B
Warfarin recommended for mechanical heart valves and target INR intensity based on type and location of prosthesis	I	B
With prior stroke, TIA, or CHA_2DS_2-VASc score ≥2, oral anticoagulants recommended. Options include:		
• Warfarin	I	A
• Dabigatran, rivaroxaban, or apixaban	I	B

Continued

Continued

Table 8: The 2014 American Heart Association/American College of Cardiology/Heart Rhythm Society guidelines for risk-based antithrombotic treatment[12]

Recommendations	CoR	LoE
With warfarin, determine INR at least weekly during initiation of therapy and monthly when stable	I	A
Direct thrombin or factor Xa inhibitor recommended if unable to maintain therapeutic INR	I	C
Reevaluate the need for anticoagulation at periodic intervals	I	C
Bridging therapy with UFH or LMWH recommended with a mechanical heart valve if warfarin is interrupted. Bridging therapy should balance risks of stroke and bleeding	I	C
For patients without mechanical heart valves, bridging therapy decisions should balance stroke and bleeding risks against duration of time patient will not be anticoagulated	I	C
Evaluate renal function before initiation of direct thrombin or factor Xa inhibitors, and reevaluate when clinically indicated and at least annually	I	B
For atrial flutter, antithrombotic therapy is recommended as for AF	I	C
With nonvalvular AF and CHA_2DS_2-VASc score of 0, it is reasonable to omit antithrombotic therapy	IIa	B
With CHA_2DS_2-VASc score ≥2 and end-stage CKD (CrCl <15 mL/min) or on hemodialysis, it is reasonable to prescribe warfarin for oral anticoagulation	IIa	B
With nonvalvular AF and a CHA_2DS_2-VASc score of 1, no antithrombotic therapy or treatment with oral anticoagulant or aspirin may be considered	IIb	C
With moderate-to-severe CKD and CHA_2DS_2-VASc scores ≥2, reduced doses of direct thrombin or factor Xa inhibitors may be considered	IIb	C
For PCI,* BMS may be considered to minimize duration of DAPT	IIb	C
After coronary revascularization in patients with CHA_2DS_2-VASc score ≥2, it may be reasonable to use clopidogrel concurrently with oral anticoagulants but without aspirin	IIb	B
Direct thrombin dabigatran and factor Xa inhibitor rivaroxaban are not recommended in patients with AF and end-stage CKD or on dialysis because of a lack of evidence from clinical trials regarding the balance of risks and benefits	III: No benefit	C
Direct thrombin inhibitor dabigatran should not be used with a mechanical heart valve	III: Harm	B

AF, atrial fibrillation; BMS, bare-metal stent; CKD, chronic kidney disease; CoR, class of recommendation; CrCl, creatinine clearance; DAPT, dualantiplatelet therapy; INR. international normalized ratio; LMWH, low-molecular-weight heparin; LoE: level of evidence; N/A, not applicable; PCI, percutaneous coronary intervention; TIA, transient ischemic attack; UFH, unfractionated heparin.

*Please see the 2011 PCI guideline for type of stent and duration of DAPT recommendations.

KEY POINTS

- Atrial fibrillation is a powerful independent risk factor for ischemic stroke
- Simple assessment tools have been developed to predict the risk of stroke ($CHADS_2$ and CHA_2DS_2-VASc scores) and bleeding (HAS-BLED score)
- Anticoagulation therapy has been associated with significant stroke risk reduction as evidenced by various randomized trials
- Anticoagulant therapy is superior to antiplatelet therapy in reducing the risk of stroke
- The superior efficacy of VKAs in stroke prevention, as evidenced in randomized trials, can be translated into clinical practice
- Several guidelines and recommendations have been established for the effective management of anticoagulant therapy and the prevention of thromboembolism in patients with AF.

REFERENCES

1. European Heart Rhythm Association; European Association for Cardio-Thoracic Surgery, Camm AJ, Kirchhof P, Lip GY, Schotten U, et al. Guidelines for the management of atrial fibrillation: the Task Force for the Management of Atrial Fibrillation of the European Society of Cardiology. Eur Heart J. 2010;31(19):2369-429.
2. Wolf PA, Abbott RD, Kannel WB. Atrial fibrillation as an independent risk factor for stroke: the Framingham Study. Stroke. 1991;22(8):983-8.
3. Gage BF, Waterman AD, Shannon W, et al. Validation of clinical classification schemes for predicting stroke: results from the National Registry of Atrial Fibrillation. JAMA. 2001;285(22):2864-70.
4. Crystal E. Role of oral anticoagulation in management of atrial fibrillation. Heart. 2004;90(7):813-7.
5. Go AS. Efficacy of anticoagulation for stroke prevention and risk stratification in atrial fibrillation: translating trials into clinical practice. Am J Manag Care. 2004;10(3 Suppl):S58-65.
6. Aguilar MI, Hart R Pearce LA. Oral anticoagulants versus antiplatelet therapy for preventing stroke in patients with nonvalvular atrial fibrillation and no history of stroke or transient ischemic attacks. Cochrane Database Syst Rev. 2007;(3):CD006186.
7. Kalra L Yu G, Perez I, Lakhani A, Donaldson N. Prospective cohort study to determine if trial efficacy of anticoagulation for stroke prevention in atrial fibrillation translates into clinical effectiveness. BMJ. 2000;320(7244):1236-9.
8. Evans A, Perez I, Yu G, Kalra L. Should stroke subtype influence anticoagulation decisions to prevent recurrence in stroke patients with atrial fibrillation? Stroke. 2001;32(12):2828-32.
9. Evans A, Perez I, Yu G, Kalra L. Secondary stroke prevention in atrial fibrillation: lessons from clinical practice. Stroke. 2000;31(9):2106-11.
10. Go A, Hylek EM, Chang Y, et al. Anticoagulation therapy for stroke prevention in atrial fibrillation: how well do randomized trials translate into clinical practice? JAMA. 2003;290(20):2685-92.
11. Camm AJ, Lip GY, De Caterina R, et al. 2012 focused update of the ESC guidelines for the management of atrial fibrillation: an update of the 2010 ESC Guidelines for the management of atrial fibrillation. Developed with the special contribution of the European Heart Rhythm Association. Eur Heart J. 2012;33(21):2719-47.
12. January CT, Wann LS, Alpert JS, et al. 2014 AHA/ACC/HRS guideline for the management of patients with atrial fibrillation: Executive summary. A report of the American College of Cardiology/American Heart Association Task Force on Practice Guidelines and the Heart Rhythm Society. Circulation. 2014;130(23):2071-2104.

9

Prevention and Management of DVT and PE and Role of Vitamin K Antagonists

Prashant Vaijyanath

INTRODUCTION

Venous thromboembolism (VTE) is a group of disorders associated with thrombus formation in the blood vessels and its consequences. It includes deep vein thrombosis (DVT) and pulmonary embolism (PE). Venous thromboembolism is significantly associated with patient morbidity and mortality. The incidence of VTE is estimated to be high in hospitalized patients (34.7%), as they are predisposed to multiple risk factors. Around 5–10% of deaths in hospitalized patients are associated with PE, making VTE the most common preventable cause of in-hospital mortality.[1] This chapter presents an overview of VTE, its risk factors, and diagnostic methods. It further focuses on the therapeutic management of VTE through anticoagulation and provides guidelines for the use of oral anticoagulants in VTE prophylaxis.

PATHOGENESIS AND CLASSIFICATION OF VENOUS THROMBOEMBOLISM

What Initiates Venous Thromboembolism?[2]

The venous valves play an essential role in aiding blood circulation to the extremities and are also known to be susceptible to stasis and hypoxia. The venous valvular sinus is believed to be the site of initiation of VTE, as indicated by direct evidence from autopsy studies. The causative factor of this phenomenon is believed to be stasis. Valvular sinus stasis is also responsible for creating a potentially hypercoagulable microenvironment associated with hypoxia and increased hematocrit. Moreover, the expression of certain vessel-based proteins, such as thrombomodulin and endothelial protein C receptor (EPCR), is sensitive to changes in the environment; hence, hypoxia or inflammation may lead to their down-regulation and the potential initiation of VTE.

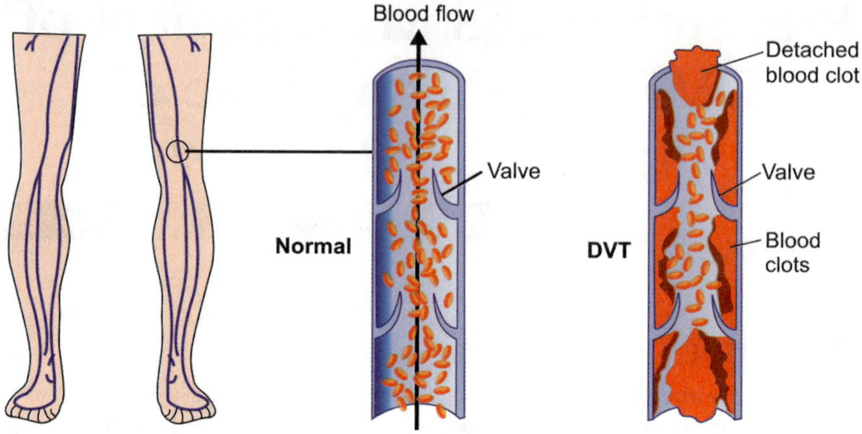

DVT, deep vein thrombosis.

Fig. 1: Pictorial depiction of leg veins

Classification of Venous Thromboembolism

Deep Venous Thrombosis

Deep venous thrombosis makes its appearance in the calf region of the leg. The majority of distal DVT is asymptomatic and is likely to resolve spontaneously. Most symptoms arise due to the extension of distal DVT into the popliteal and femoral veins and other proximal veins (Fig. 1). There is a 60–70% chance of DVT development in patients with symptomatic VTE. Complications of DVT include post-phlebitic syndrome, PE, and death. Around 50% of untreated symptomatic proximal DVT may lead to symptomatic PE within 3 months. Post-thrombotic syndrome is another serious complication of DVT, occurring in 20–50% of patients and resulting in lifelong limb pain, inflammation, edema, and leg ulcers. Severe post-thrombotic syndrome may result in DVT recurrence in 10% of patients within 5 years.[3]

Pulmonary Embolism

Around 30–40% of VTE patients may exhibit symptoms associated with PE (new or worsening dyspnea, chest pain, sustained hypotension). Since the initial clinical presentation in 25% of such patients is sudden death, PE is associated with a much lower survival rate than DVT. In patients not undergoing further treatment, the PE fatality rate can be as high as 25%. The prescription of anticoagulant treatment could, however, reduce this risk to 1.5%.[3]

Risk Factors for Venous Thromboembolism

An understanding of the predisposing factors for VTE is required for the effective management of the disease in high-risk patients. The major and minor risk factors of VTE are listed in table 1.[4]

Table 1: Major and minor risk factors for venous thromboembolism[4]

Major risk factors (relative risk 5–20)	
Surgery*	• Major abdominal/pelvic surgery • Hip/knee replacement • Postoperative intensive care
Obstetrics	• Late pregnancy • Cesarean section • Puerperium
Lower limb problems	• Fracture • Varicose veins
Malignancy	• Abdominal/pelvic • Advanced/metastatic
Reduced mobility	• Hospitalization • Institutional care
Miscellaneous	Previous proven VTE
Minor risk factors (relative risk 2–4)	
Cardiovascular	• Congenital heart disease • Congestive cardiac failure • Hypertension • Superficial venous thrombosis • Indwelling central vein catheter
Estrogens	• Oral contraceptive • Hormone replacement therapy
Miscellaneous	• COPD • Neurological disability • Occult malignancy • Thrombotic disorders • Long distance sedentary travel • Obesity • Other†

COPD, chronic obstructive pulmonary disease.
*Where appropriate prophylaxis is used, relative risk is much lower.
†Inflammatory bowel disease, nephrotic syndrome, chronic dialysis, myeloproliferative disorders, paroxysmal nocturnal hemoglobinuria, Behçet's disease.

Venous thromboembolism occurs due to the cumulative effects of endogenous, genetic, and environmental risk factors (Fig. 2).[5]

Clinical Prediction of Deep Vein Thrombosis[6]

Clinical Model for Predicting Pretest Probability of Deep Vein Thrombosis (Wells Score)

A clinical model developed by the standardization of clinical assessment, based on a combination of risk factors, signs and symptoms, and the subsequent stratification of patients suspected of DVT, is the most

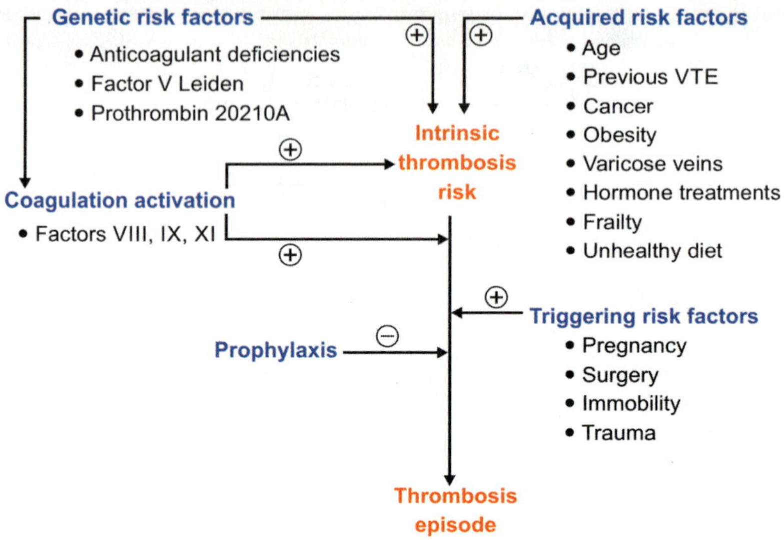

VTE, venous thromboembolism.

Fig. 2: Interaction between risk factors in the development of venous thromboembolism[5]

Table 2: Pretest probability assessment of deep vein thrombosis (Wells score)[6]

	Points
Active cancer (treatment ongoing or within previous 6 months or palliative)	1
Paralysis, paresis, or recent plaster immobilization of the lower extremities	1
Recently bedridden for 3 days or major surgery within 12 weeks requiring general or regional anesthesia	1
Localized tenderness along the distribution of the deep veins	1
Entire leg swollen	1
Calf swelling 3 cm, asymptomatic side (measured 10 cm below tibial tuberosity)	1
Pitting edema limited to the symptomatic leg	1
Collateral superficial veins (nonvaricose)	1
Previous DVT	1
Alternative diagnosis as likely as or more likely than DVT	-2
Notes: DVT unlikely: ≤1; DVT likely: ≥2	

commonly accepted evidence-based strategy for diagnosing VTE. The most recommended model by Wells et al. stratifies patients into two risk categories: "DVT unlikely" (clinical score <1) and "DVT likely" (clinical score >1) (Table 2).

Diagnostic Algorithm using D-Dimer Testing and Ultrasound

A diagnostic algorithm based on the Wells score, D-dimer (degradation product of cross-linked fibrin and best-recognized biomarker for initial suspected VTE) assay, and venous ultrasonography has been developed for patients with suspected DVT (Flowchart. 1).

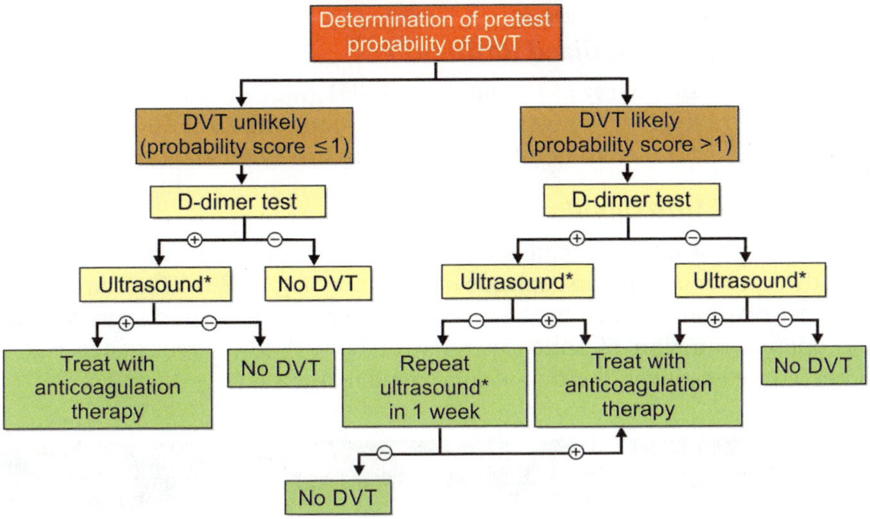

DVT, deep vein thrombosis.

Flowchart 1: Diagnostic algorithm using D-dimer testing and ultrasound[6]

*Imagine done from proximal veins of calf trifurcation.

Imaging in Suspected Deep Vein Thrombosis Patients

Magnetic resonance imaging (MRI) is highly sensitive in detecting calf and pelvic DVT as well as upper extremity venous thromboses. MRIs can be used to rule out other conditions in suspected DVT patients.

Management of Deep Vein Thrombosis and Pulmonary Embolism

The major therapeutic goal in the management of VTE is the prevention of the local extension and subsequent embolization of thrombus and, in certain clinical cases, also the acceleration of fibrinolysis.[7]

Role of Anticoagulation in Venous Thromboembolism[7]

Anticoagulants prevent clinically important thrombus extension and are considered effective in the majority of patients. Heparin and coumarins are the most commonly used anticoagulants, which, when administered in low doses, inhibit the production of factor Xa and thrombin. The mode of action of oral anticoagulants does not involve the direct inhibition of thrombin, but rather the modulation of further thrombin generation by the reduction of functional coagulation factors involved in the positive feedback loop. Anticoagulation therapy is effective in VTE patients and prevents progression to PE. Evidence suggests a high rate of mortality and recurrence in untreated PE patients, as well as high recurrence rates in untreated patients with symptomatic proximal or calf-vein thrombosis. Anticoagulation aids in reducing recurrence in DVT patients and is also beneficial in reducing mortality and recurrence in patients with acute PE.

Recommended Therapeutic International Normalized Ratio ranges[8]

As per the British Society of Hematology (BSH) guidelines, the international normalized ratio (INR) ranges to be maintained with oral anticoagulation therapy in various thromboembolic conditions are listed in table 3.

Duration of Anticoagulation

The duration of anticoagulant therapy depends on whether the patient has already experienced the first episode of DVT; ongoing VTE risk factors; and the presence of thrombophlebitis.[6] Several studies have been conducted to evaluate the optimal duration of anticoagulation therapy. A lower recurrence risk is observed with a longer duration of anticoagulant therapy (Figs 3 and 4).[9,10]

Table 3: Therapeutic international normalized ratio range to be maintained with anticoagulant therapy[8]

INR	Clinical state
2.0–2.5	• Prophylaxis of deep vein thrombosis including surgery on high-risk patients • (2.0–3.0 for hip surgery and fractured femur operations)
2.0–3.0	• Treatment of deep vein thrombosis • Pulmonary embolism • Systemic embolism • Prevention of venous thromboembolism in myocardial infarction • Mitral stenosis with embolism • Transient ischemic attacks • Atrial fibrillation
3.0–4.5	• Recurrent deep vein thrombosis and pulmonary embolism • Arterial disease including myocardial infarction • Mechanical prosthetic heart valves

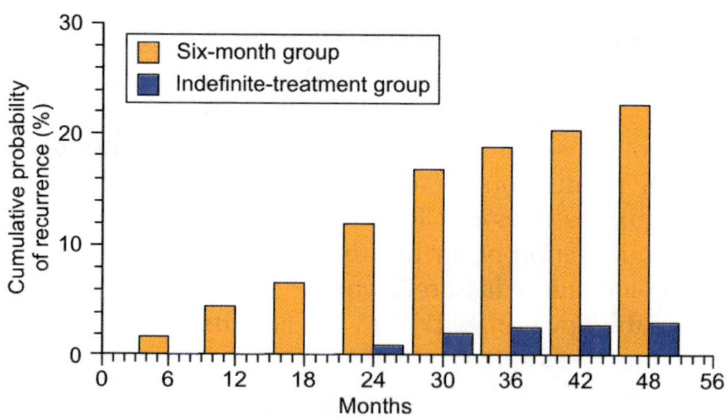

Fig. 3: Cumulative probability of recurrent venous thromboembolism in patients after a second episode of thromboembolic event, with respect to the duration of anticoagulant therapy[9]

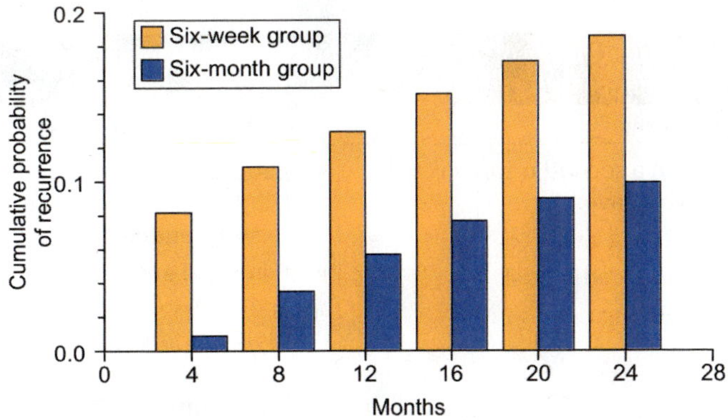

Fig. 4: Cumulative probability of recurrent venous thromboembolism in patients after a first episode of thromboembolic event, with respect to the duration of anticoagulant therapy[10]

Vitamin K antagonists are known to be highly effective in reducing the recurrence rates of VTE during treatment, but they do not eliminate the risk of VTE after discontinuation of therapy. Thus, the duration of vitamin K antagonists (VKA) treatment in a particular patient depends more on the estimated risk of recurrence after discontinuation than the risk of bleeding complications while on treatment.[11]

The duration of anticoagulant treatment as per the American College of Chest Physicians (ACCP) 2016 guidelines is summarized in table 4.[12]

Table 4: American College of Chest Physicians guidelines for duration of anticoagulant treatment[12]

Patient indication	Recommendation
• Patients with a proximal DVT of the leg or PE provoked by surgery	• Treatment with anticoagulation for 3 months
• Patients with a proximal DVT of the leg or PE provoked by a nonsurgical transient risk factor • Patients with low, moderate, or high risk of bleeding	• Treatment with anticoagulation for 3 months
• Patients with an isolated distal DVT of the leg provoked by surgery or a nonsurgical transient risk factor	• Treatment with anticoagulation for 3 months
• Patients with an unprovoked DVT of the leg (isolated distal or proximal) or PE	• Treatment with anticoagulation for 3 months
• Patients with a first VTE that is an unprovoked proximal DVT of the leg or PE and who have: o Low or moderate bleeding risk o High bleeding risk	• Extended anticoagulant therapy (no scheduled stop date) is recommended over 3 months of therapy • 3 months of anticoagulant therapy is recommended over extended therapy (no scheduled stop date)

Continued

Continued

Table 4: American College of Chest Physicians guidelines for duration of anticoagulant treatment[12]

Patient indication	Recommendation
• Patients with a second unprovoked VTE and who have: o Low bleeding risk o Moderate bleeding risk o High bleeding risk	• Extended anticoagulant therapy (no scheduled stop date) is recommended over 3 months • Extended anticoagulant therapy is recommended over 3 months of therapy • 3 months of anticoagulant therapy is recommended over extended therapy (no scheduled stop date)
• In patients with DVT of the leg or PE and active cancer (cancer-associated thrombosis) and who: o Do not have a high bleeding risk o Have a high bleeding risk	• Extended anticoagulant therapy (no scheduled stop date) is recommended over 3 months

DVT, deep vein thrombosis; PE, pulmonary embolism; VTE, venous thromboembolism.

Prevention of Venous Thromboembolism Recurrence

A number of factors may lead to the recurrence of VTE. These factors may be linked to the thrombotic event itself or to patient characteristics and conditions (Table 5).[13]

The need for long-term anticoagulation to prevent recurrent episodes of VTE has been supported by several studies. A study that included patients with symptomatic calf-vein thrombosis showed a significantly higher rate of recurrence (68%) in patients not receiving oral anticoagulant therapy compared to those receiving anticoagulant therapy (5%), in 1 year.[14]

Table 5: Risk factors for recurrence of venous thromboembolism after a first event[13]

Thrombosis related	Patient related
• Unprovoked event • Nonsurgical transient versus surgical risk factor associated with the first event • Proximal (especially if iliofemoral) versus distal DVT • Pulmonary embolism • Persistence of residual vein thrombosis	• Men • Active cancer • Antiphospholipid syndrome • Inherited thrombophilic alterations • Pregnancy and puerperium • Hormonal therapies • Obesity • Presence of inferior vena cava filter • Polycythemia vera and essential thrombocythemia, especially in the presence of JAK2 V617F mutation

DVT, deep vein thrombosis

A randomized study conducted in 4,289 patients with symptomatic VTE evaluated the efficacy of different VKAs in the prevention of recurrent VTE events. The study reported that the recurrence of DVT was lower with acenocoumarol than with warfarin (Fig. 5).[15]

Vitamin K antagonists are used in the standard therapy for long-term secondary prophylaxis. Oral anticoagulation therapy may be needed for more than 3 months. The decision to continue oral anticoagulation therapy beyond 3 months depends on the following factors:[16]

- Risk of recurrent thrombosis and anticoagulant-related bleeding
- Patient preference.

Prophylaxis of Venous Thromboembolism in High Risk Patients

Certain groups of patients are at high risk of developing VTE. Such patients include surgical patients (orthopedic surgery, neurosurgery, gynecological surgery, and others), medically ill patients, and patients with conditions that provoke VTE (such as pregnancy and cancer).

Successful prevention strategies for different levels of VTE risk in surgical patients not receiving prophylaxis are listed in table 6.[17]

A prospective study evaluated the efficacy and safety of acenocoumarol in 39 critically ill neurological patients requiring prolonged mechanical ventilation. The study revealed that acenocoumarol was as effective as other anticoagulants in the prevention of DVT in the critically ill.[18]

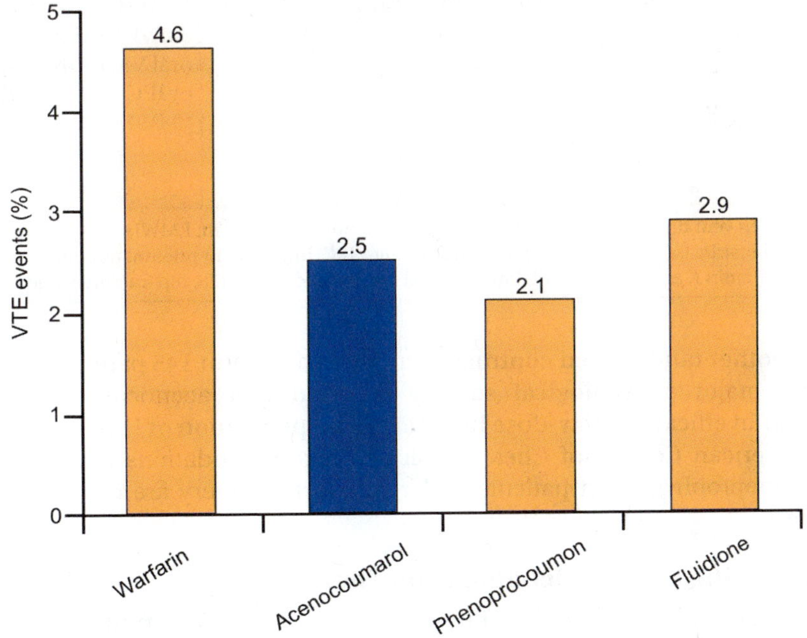

Fig. 5: Efficacy of vitamin K antagonists in the prevention of venous thromboembolism[15]

Table 6: Risk of venous thromboembolism in surgical patients not receiving any prophylaxis and corresponding prevention stratergies[17]

Level of risk	DVT (%)		PE (%)		Successful prevention strategies
	Calf	Proximal	Clinical	Fatal	
Low risk					
Minor surgery inpatients <40 years with no additional risk factors	2	0.4	0.2	< 0.01	No specific prophylaxis; early and aggressive mobilization
Moderate risk					
Minor surgery in patients with additional risk factors Surgery in patients aged 40 to 60 years with no additional risk factors	10–20	2–4	1–2	0.1–0.4	LDUH (q12h), LMWH (≤3400 U daily), GCS, or IPC
High risk					
Surgery in patients >60 years, or 40–60 years with additional risk factors	20–40	4–8	2–4	0.4–1.0	LDUH (q8h), LMWH (>3400 U daily), or IPC
Highest risk					
Surgery in patients with multiple risk factors Hip or knee arthroplasty, HFS Major trauma; spinal cord injury	40–80	10–20	4–10	0.2–5.0	LMWH (>3400 U daily), fondaparinux oral VKAs (INR 2–3), or IPC/GCS+LDUH/ LMWH

DVT, deep vein thrombosis; LDUH, low-dose unfractionated heparin; LMWH, low-molecular-weight heparin; GCS, graded compression stockings; IPC, intermittent pneumatic compression; VKAs, vitamin K antagonists, INR, international normalized ratio; HFS, hip fracture surgery.

Another randomized controlled study conducted in 145 patients undergoing major gynecological surgery reported that acenocoumarol was similar in efficacy to low-dose heparin, in the prevention of DVT (Fig. 6).[19]

American College of Chest Physicians recommendations for choosing thromboprophylaxis in patients undergoing orthosurgery are mentioned in table 7.[20]

Monitoring Oral Anticoagulation Therapy

American College of Chest Physicians guidelines recommend that in patients treated with VKAs, the INR should be maintained between 2.0

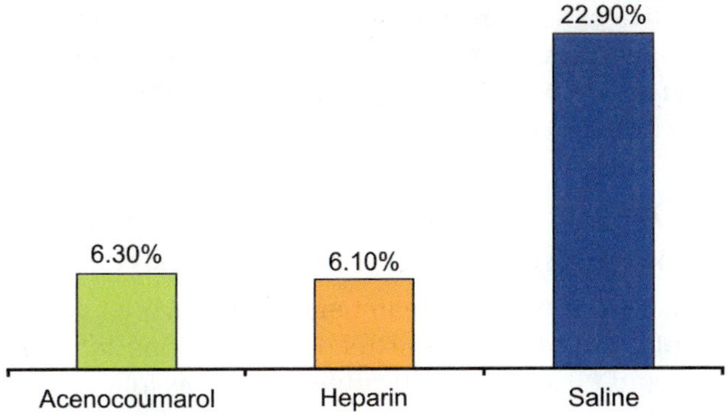

Fig. 6: Efficacy of acenocoumarol and low-dose heparin in the prevention of deep vein thrombosis in patients undergoing gynecological surgery[19]

Table 7: American College of Chest Physicians recommendations for choosing thromboprophylaxis in orthopedic surgery patients[20]

Type of orthopedic surgery	Recommended anticoagulants
Hip fracture surgery	VKA, LMWH, fondaparinux, low-dose UFH, aspirin, or intermittent pneumatic device (ICPD) for a minimum of 10–15 days
Total hip arthroplasty/total knee arthroplasty	VKA, LMWH, fondaparinux, low-dose UFH, apixaban, dabigatran, rivaroxaban, aspirin, or IPCD for a minimum of 10–15 days

VKA, vitamin K antagonists; LMWH, low molecular weight heparin; UFH, unfractionated heparin

and 3.0 (target INR: 2.5). For patients taking VKA therapy with consistently stable INRs, an INR testing frequency of up to 12 weeks rather than every 4 weeks is recommended.[21]

Special Conditions

Pregnancy

Pulmonary embolism is the leading cause of pregnancy-related deaths. The risk is particularly higher in the postpartum period, especially after cesarean section. Heparin and its analogs are recommended in pregnant women, as these do not cross the placenta. However, after delivery, switching over to VKAs may be suggested, as they are safe in lactating women. It is recommended to continue anticoagulants for at least 3 months after delivery.[4,11]

Cancer Patients

Cancer is a major risk factor for the recurrence of VTE events. The risk of thrombosis among cancer patients is fourfold higher than in the general population. The risk further increases to about six- or sevenfold in patients receiving chemotherapy. This may be attributed to the risk of thrombotic events, typically associated with a large number of anticancer drugs. Thus, patients with active cancer are suitable candidates for an indefinite duration of anticoagulation therapy. In cancer patients, LMWH should be initiated and continued for the first 3–6 months, followed by either LMWH or VKA up to an indefinite duration or until the cancer is treated.[4]

ANTITHROMBOTIC THERAPY FOR VENOUS THROMBOEMBOLISM: SUMMARY OF GUIDELINES

Several groups of experts and researchers have provided guidelines for the management of PE and DVT. The recommendations for anticoagulation therapy in DVT and PE as per ACCP guidelines are as follows (Table 8):[22]

Table 8: Recommendations for anticoagulation therapy in deep vein thrombosis and pulmonary embolism[22]

Patient indication	Recommendation
Patients with acute DVT of the leg treated with VKA therapy	Initial treatment with parenteral anticoagulation (low-molecular-weight heparin, fondaparinux, IV, UFH, or SC, UFH)
Patients with a high and intermediate clinical suspicion of acute VTE	Treatment with parenteral anticoagulants while awaiting results of the diagnostic tests
Patients with acute isolated distal DVT or acute proximal DVT of the leg and severe symptoms or risk factors for extension	Initial anticoagulation therapy recommended
Patients with acute isolated distal DVT of the leg who are managed with serial imaging	Anticoagulation therapy recommended if the thrombus extends to distal or proximal veins
In patients with acute DVT of the leg	Early initiation of VKA over delayed initiation is recommended usually the same day as parenteral therapy initiation. Parenteral anticoagulation should be continued for a minimum of 5 days and until the international normalized ratio is ≥2.0 for at least 24 h. The use of inferior vena cava filter, in addition to anticoagulant therapy, is not recommended.
Patients with acute proximal DVT of the leg	Anticoagulant therapy alone is recommended over catheter-directed thrombolysis, systemic thrombolysis, and operative venous thrombectomy
Patients with acute PE	Initial treatment with parenteral anticoagulation (low-molecular-weight heparin, fondaparinux, IV, UFH, or SC, UFH)

Continued

Continued

Table 8: Recommendations for anticoagulation therapy in deep vein thrombosis and pulmonary embolism[22]

Patient indication	Recommendation
Patients with a high and intermediate clinical suspicion of acute PE	Treatment with parenteral anticoagulants while awaiting results of the diagnostic tests
Patients with acute PE	Early initiation of VKA over delayed initiation is recommended usually the same day as parenteral therapy initiation. Parenteral anticoagulation should be continued for a minimum of 5 days and until the international normalized ratio is ≥2.0 for at least 24 h.

DVT, deep vein thrombosis; VKA, vitamin K antagonists; IV, intravenous; PE, pulmonary embolism; UFH, unfractionated heparin; SC, subcutaneous.

KEY POINTS

- Venous thromboembolism, classified into DVT and PE, is a major cause of morbidity and mortality, especially in hospitalized patients
- Understanding the risk factors for VTE is essential for the effective management of the condition
- Several diagnostic strategies for VTE have been developed, such as the Wells pretest probability model and the D-dimer and ultrasound algorithm
- Anticoagulants prevent thrombus extension and are considered an effective prophylactic therapy in patients with VTE
- Long-term anticoagulant treatment is beneficial and has been associated with fewer cases of recurrence of VTE
- Monitoring VKA therapy and the maintenance of therapeutic INR are essential for effective treatment without any therapy-related complications
- The use of anticoagulant therapy is advantageous in patients with a high risk of VTE, as well as in special population groups
- Guidelines have been proposed to aid clinicians in the successful management of antithrombotic therapy in VTE.

REFERENCES

1. API India. (2010). Venous thromboembolism—Indian perspective. [online] Available from http://www.apiindia.org/pdf/medicine_update_2010/cardiology_31.pdf. [Accessed February, 2017].
2. Esmon CT. Basic mechanisms and pathogenesis of venous thrombosis. Blood Rev. 2009;23(5):225-9.
3. Moheimani F, Jackson D. Venous thromboembolism: Classification, risk factors, diagnosis, and management. ISRN Hematology. 2011;2011:1-7.
4. British Thoracic Society Standards of Care Committee Pulmonary Embolism Guideline Development Group. British Thoracic Society guidelines for the management of suspected acute pulmonary embolism. Thorax. 2003;58(6):470-83.

5. Cushman M. Epidemiology and risk factors for venous thrombosis. Semi hematol. 2007;44(2):62-9.
6. Kesieme E, Kesieme C, Jebbin N, Irekpita E, Dongo A. Deep vein thrombosis: a clinical review. J Blood Med. 2011;2(2):59-69.
7. Hirsh J, Hoak J. Management of deep vein thrombosis and pulmonary embolism a statement for healthcare professionals from the Council on Thrombosis (in Consultation with the Council on Cardiovascular Radiology). J Am Heart Assoc. 1996;93(12):2212-45.
8. Guidelines on oral anticoagulation: second edition. British Society for Haematology. British Committee for Standards in Haematology. Haemostasis and Thrombosis Task Force. J Clin Path. 1990;43(3):177-83.
9. Schulman S, Granqvist S, Holmström M, Carlsson A, Lindmarker P, Nicol P, et al. The duration of oral anticoagulant therapy after a second episode of venous thromboembolism. The Duration of Anticoagulation Trial Study Group. N Engl J Med. 1997;336(6):393-8.
10. Schulman S, Rhedin AS, Lindmarker P, Carlsson A, Lärfars G, Nicol P, et al. A comparison of six weeks with six months of oral anticoagulant therapy after a first episode of venous thromboembolism. Duration of Anticoagulation Trial Study Group. N Engl J Med. 1995;332(25):1661-5.
11. Guidelines on the diagnosis and management of acute pulmonary embolism: the Task Force for the Diagnosis and Management of Acute Pulmonary Embolism of the European Society of Cardiology (ESC). Eur Heart J. 2008;29(18):2276-315.
12. Kearon C, Akl EA, Ornelas J, Blaivas A, Jimenez D, Bounameaux H, et al. Antithrombotic Therapy for VTE Disease: CHEST Guideline and Expert Panel Report. Chest. 2016; 149(2):315-52.
13. Palareti G. Recurrent venous thromboembolism: What is the risk and how to prevent it. Scientifica. 2012;2012:1-17.
14. Lagerstedt CI, Olsson CG, Fagher B, Oqvist BW, Albrechtsson U. Need for long-term anticoagulant treatment in symptomatic calf-vein thrombosis. Lancet. 1985;2(8454):515-8.
15. Lensing AWA. Efficacy and safety of various vitamin K antagonists for the treatment of symptomatic venous thromboembolism. Hematol Meet Rep. 2008;2:11-2.
16. Mahapatra M, Mishra P, Seth T, Saxena R. Medical management of deep vein thrombosis. East J Med. 2009;14(2):69-72.
17. Caprini JA. (2005). Risk factors of venous thromboembolism. The American Journal of Medicine UPDATE. [online] Available from http://www.venousdisease.com/Publications/Update%20on%20risk%20factors-caprini.pdf. [Accessed February, 2016].
18. Azim A, Baronia AK, Rao BP, Singh RK, Gurjar M, Singh N. Safety and cost-effectiveness of acitrom for DVT prophylaxis in critically ill patients requiring prolonged mechanical ventilation—A preliminary experience. J Anaesthesiol Clin Pharmacol. 2010;26(3):360-2.
19. Taberner DA, Poller L, Burslem RW, Jones JB. Oral anticoagulants controlled by the British comparative thromboplastin versus low-dose heparin in prophylaxis of deep vein thrombosis. Br Med J. 1978;1:272-4.
20. Guyatt GH, Akl EA, Crowther M, Gutterman DD, Schuünemann HJ; American College of Chest Physicians Antithrombotic Therapy and Prevention of Thrombosis Panel. Executive Summary: Antithrombotic Therapy and Prevention of Thrombosis, 9th ed: American College of Chest Physicians Evidence-Based Clinical Practice Guidelines. Chest. 2012; 141(2):7S-47S.
21. Holbrook A, Schulman S, Witt DM, Vandvik PO, Fish J, Kovacs MJ, et al. Evidence-based management of anticoagulation therapy: Antithrombotic therapy and prevention of thrombosis, 9th ed: American College of Chest Physicians Evidence-Based Clinical Practice Guidelines. Chest. 2012;141(2 Suppl):e152S-84S.
22. Kearon C, Akl EA, Comerota AJ, Prandoni P, Bounameaux H, Goldhaber SZ, et al. Antithrombotic therapy for VTE disease: Antithrombotic therapy and prevention of thrombosis: American College of Chest Physicians evidence-based clinical practice guidelines. Chest. 2012;141(2 Suppl):e419S-94S.

10

Anticoagulation in Valvular Heart Disease

Nitin S Patki

INTRODUCTION

Valvular heart disease (VHD) encompasses a variety of cardiovascular conditions and accounts for 10–20% of all cardiac surgical procedures.[1] It is a significant global contributor to morbidity and mortality.[2] This chapter provides an overview of VHD and its therapeutic management through oral anticoagulation therapy; it also focuses on the use of vitamin K antagonists in various indications of VHD and the role of acenocoumarol. The chapter further provides an overview of current guidelines for VHD management.

VALVULAR HEART DISEASE: AN OVERVIEW

Valvular heart diseases include both acquired and congenital lesions. These lesions may occur isolated or in combination with other heart conditions. Two major mechanisms might contribute to deformed cardiac valves:

1. First, an obstruction (stenosis) and/or regurgitation (incompetence) leading to increased hemodynamic load on the cardiac chambers
2. Second, infective endocarditis caused due to increased susceptibility of abdominal valves to infections.[1]

Major Valvular Lesions[3]

- Mitral regurgitation: It characterized by volume overload of the left ventricle and left atrium; in more severe cases, this may result in a progressive decline in systolic contractile function
- Mitral stenosis: It involves the progressive obstruction of left ventricular inflow due to fibrosis and partial fusion of the mitral valve leaflets
- Aortic regurgitation: It characterized by left ventricular volume overload and increased left ventricular end diastolic volume, eventually leading to left ventricular contractile dysfunction in more severe cases
- Aortic stenosis: It results from fibrosis and fusion of the valve cusps, causing progressive obstruction to left ventricular outflow.

INCIDENCE: GLOBAL AND INDIAN SCENARIO

Globally, the incidence of VHD is less common in industrialized countries compared to developing countries, where degenerative valvular disease is more prominent; however, in developing countries such as India, rheumatic fever and rheumatic heart disease (RHD) remain a huge heath care burden in both children and adults.[2] The incidence of rheumatic fever in developed countries is 0.5/100,000 population, and the prevalence is less than 0.05/1,000; comparatively, in India, RHD is estimated to affect 2–11/1,000 school children, with an average adult prevalence ranging between 123 and 200/100,000 population.[4] Rheumatic heart disease accounts for nearly 25–45% of all acquired heart diseases in India.[2]

Atrial Fibrillation and Valvular Heart Disease

Valvular heart diseases, especially left-sided valvular lesions, are frequently complicated by the presence of atrial fibrillation (AF). Aortic or mitral valve disease causes structural changes to the left atrium resulting from left atrial pressure and/or volume overload; alternatively, changes in arterial electrophysiology may ensue as a consequence of chronic arterial stretch-related fibrotic changes. Together, these developments contribute to the development of arterial arrhythmia (Fig. 1).[5]

About 30–40% of patients with mitral stenosis develop AF. The condition is associated with a poor prognosis, with a 10-year survival rate of nearly 25% compared to 46% in patients with normal sinus rhythm.[4] The prevalence of AF in patients with mitral regurgitation is also seen frequently regardless of the underlying valvular pathology. In a study involving patients with mitral regurgitation due to flail leaflets, AF was observed in 18% and 48% of patients at 5- and 10-year follow-up, respectively.[6]

Atrial Fibrillation and the Risk of Stroke

Patients with mitral heart disease are at an increased risk of adverse events, including the risk of mortality associated with atrial arrhythmias.

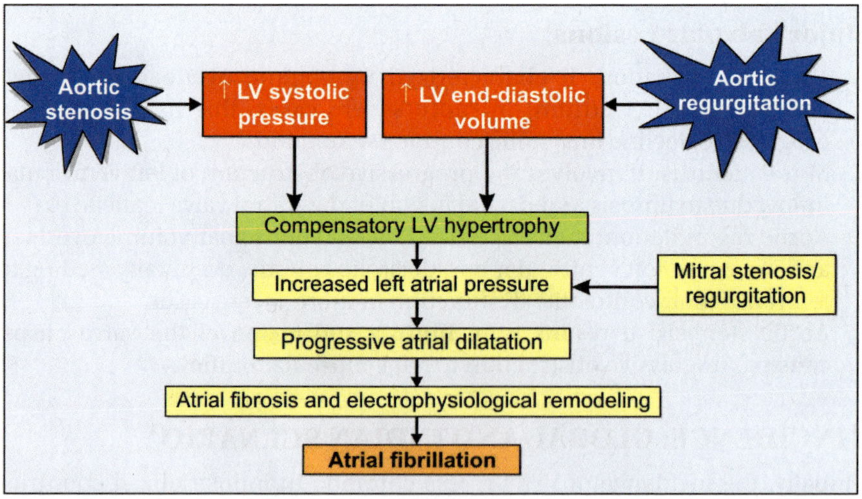

Fig. 1: Relationship between valvular heart disease and atrial fibrillation[5]

This is due to the higher prevalence of stroke in patients with mitral valve disease who develop AF.[5] In the Framingham Heart Study, a 17-fold higher risk of stroke was observed in patients with RHD and AF as compared to age-matched controls. Further, the risk was five times higher compared to those with nonrheumatic AF.[7] Around two-thirds of patients with valvular AF (mitral stenosis) who have experienced an ischemic stroke have a high probability of experiencing a second stroke in the subsequent decade, with half of them recurring as early as in the first year.[8]

As per a retrospective study, patients with rheumatic mitral stenosis in sinus rhythm with an embolic event incidence rate of 8% per year showed a significant increase in incidence rate (31.5%) with concomitant AF. Patients with rheumatic mitral regurgitation were also at an increased risk for a cardioembolic event; even among those in sinus rhythm, who had an incidence of 7.7% per year, an increase to 22% was seen in those with concomitant AF.[9]

Need for Oral Anticoagulation in Valvular Heart Disease

Indications of Vitamin K Antagonists in Valvular Heart Disease and Target International Normalized Ratio

Oral anticoagulants have been the mainstay of cardiovascular therapy in that vitamin K antagonists (VKAs) with their dose-dependent anticoagulant properties have been at the forefront of therapeutic management of heart-related diseases since the early 1950s. In fact, VKAs were the only available option for long-term use for over 60 years. Although newer oral coagulants are making their mark in patients with non-valvular AF, VKAs still remain the agent of choice for rheumatic valvular disease-associated AF and in patients with mechanical heart valves.[10]

The therapeutic advantages of antithrombotic treatment in mitigating risk of thromboembolism in valvular diseases outweigh the risk of therapy-associated bleeding complications. Several recommendations provide the international normalized ratio (INR) target range for a variety of patient indications so as to maintain an optimal balance and avoid any therapy-associated adverse events. Table 1 provides recommended INR target for specific patient conditions as per the American College of Chest Physicians (ACCP) guidelines.[11]

Recommended International Normalized Ratio for Patients with Mechanical Heart Valves

The intensity of anticoagulant treatment in patients with prosthetic mechanical valves depends on:

- The thrombogenicity of the prosthesis
- The position of the valve (aortic or mitral/tricuspid/pulmonary)
- Associated thromboembolic risk factors.

The European Society of Cardiology (ESC) recommendations for target INR in patients with mechanical valves, taking into account the intracardiac conditions and prosthesis thrombogenicity, are summarized in table 2.[10]

Table 1: American College of Chest Physicians-recommended international normalized ratio target values for patients with specific heart conditions[11]

Patient indication	Recommended target INR
Patients with rheumatic mitral valve disease and normal sinus rhythm with a left atrial diameter >55 mm	2.5
Patients with rheumatic mitral valve disease complicated by the presence of left atrial thrombus	2.5
Patients with rheumatic mitral valve disease complicated by the presence of atrial fibrillation and/or previous systemic embolism	2.5
Patients with a bioprosthetic valve in the mitral position	2.5
Patients with a mechanical aortic valve	2.5

INR, international normalized ratio.

Table 2: The European Society of Cardiology-recommended international normalized ratio targets for patients with prosthetic mechanical valves[10]

	Prosthesis thrombogenicity (as determined by valve thrombosis rates)		
In patients with prosthetic mechanical valves	**Low** [Medtronic Hall, St. Jude Medical (without Silzone), Carbomedics aortic valve replacement, bioprosthesis]	**Medium** (Bileaflet valves with insufficient data, Bjork-Shiley Valves)	**High** (Lillehei Kaster, Omniscience, Starr Edwards)
Without risk factors: • Sinus rhythm • Left atrium <50 mm • Mitral valve gradient 0 • Left ventricle-Normal • Spontaneous echo contrast 0 • Aortic valve replacement	2.5	3.0	3.5
With risk factors: • Atrial fibrillation • Left atrium >50 mm • Mitral valve gradient + • Ejection fraction <35% • Spontaneous echo contrast+ • Mitral valve replacement; tricuspid valve replacement; pulmonary valve replacement	3.0	3.5	4.0*

*There is considerable uncertainty in recommending such high-intensity anticoagulation in this group.

Box 1: Absolute indications for indefinite anticoagulant therapy[12]

Patients with mechanical prostheses:

Chronic or intermittent atrial fibrillation in the presence of

- Native valve disease
- Bioprostheses
- Valve repair
- Valvuloplastry

Patients with native valve disease and previous emboli:

Mitral valve stenosis, independent of rhythm, with

- High valve gradients
- Thrombus in left atrium
- Spontaneous echo contrast in left atrium
- Large left atrium >50 mm
- Low cardiac output
- Congestive heart failure

Absolute Indications for Lifelong Anticoagulant Therapy

Certain VHD indications, such as patient use of mechanical prosthetic valves, may warrant lifelong oral anticoagulation (Box 1).[12]

Vitamin K Antagonists for the Prevention of Thromboembolic Events in Native Valvular Heart Disease

Thromboembolic events contribute to a significant proportion of morbidity and mortality in patients with native heart valve disease and artificial heart valves. These complications can be significantly reduced by the use of oral anticoagulants.[13] Anticoagulation therapy with vitamin K antagonists (VKAs) is strongly indicated for patients with AF associated with RHD, prosthetic mitral valves of any type, or a previous embolism [stroke or transient ischemic attack (TIA)].[14]

The intensity of oral anticoagulant treatment in VHDs must take into account the risk factors for thromboembolic events. Patients with mitral stenosis have the highest risk for thromboembolism; this is particularly so in those with concomitant AF, in such case the risk of thromboembolism increases up to 20% annually. An 18-fold increase in embolic risk is associated with AF-related mitral valve disease. Other risk factors include reduced ventricular function and cardiac output, cardiac heart failure, and left atrial enlargement. A loss in atrial contraction also carries an increased risk of thromboembolism despite an electrophysiologically normal sinus rhythm. The degree of mitral stenosis is also an important embolic risk factor. Severe mitral stenosis is susceptible to embolism regardless of the presence of sinus rhythm. A 20% recurrence rate is associated with a history of previous peripheral emboli.[12]

Oral Anticoagulation in Patients with Mitral Valve Prolapse[15]

Mitral valve prolapse (MPV) is the most common form of valve disease in adults. There have been reports of an association between MVP and stroke.

Table 3: Recommendations for oral anticoagulation in patients with mitral valve prolapse[15]

Patients subgroup	ACCP grading recommendation
In people with MVP who have not experienced systemic embolism, unexplained TIAs, or AF, ACCP recommends against any antithrombotic therapy	Grade IC
In patients with MVP who have documented but unexplained TIAs, long-term aspirin therapy, 50–162 mg/day is recommended	Grade IA
In patients with MVP who have documented systemic embolism or recurrent TIAs despite aspirin therapy, long-term vitamin K antagonist therapy (target INR, 2.5; range 2.0–3.0) is recommended	Grade 2C

ACCP, American College of Chest Physicians; MPV, Mitral valve prolapse; TIAs, transient ischemic attacks; AF, atrial fibrillation; INR, international normalized ratio

A study indicated that among 60 patients aged less than 45 years who had a TIA or stroke, 40% had MVP. The Seventh ACCP recommendations on oral anticoagulation for patients with MVP are listed in table 3.[15]

Oral Anticoagulation in Patients with Mitral Annular Calcification[15]

Mitral annular calcification (MAC)-associated thromboembolism may result from several factors, such as:

- Presence of AF
- Mitral valve lesion-related hemodynamic consequences (stenosis and regurgitation)
- Fragmentation of calcific annular tissue
- Diffuse vascular atherosclerosis.

Anticoagulation for Patients with Aortic Valve and Aortic Arch Disorder

The occurrence of clinically detectable systemic emboli in isolated aortic valve (AV) disease is rare. Systemic embolism in patients with AV disease is also uncommon in the absence of associated mitral valve disease or AF, but microscopic calcific emboli can be seen in those with severe calcific AV disease. The Seventh ACCP recommendations on oral anticoagulation for patients with AV and AAD are presented in table 4.[15]

Infective Endocarditis and Anticoagulation[15]

A decrease in the incidence of systemic emboli in infective endocarditis has been noted with effective antibiotic use. Emboli occur more frequently in patients with acute endocarditis than in those with subacute disease. The incidence of pulmonary emboli in right-sided endocarditis is particularly high. The seventh ACCP recommendations on oral anticoagulation for patients with endocarditis are listed in table 5.

Table 4: Recommendations for oral anticoagulation in patients with mitral annular calcification[15]	
Patients subgroup	**ACCP grading recommendation**
In patients with MAC complicated by systemic embolism, not documented to be calcific embolism, treatment with long-term OAC therapy with a target INR of 2.5 (INR range, 2.0–3.0) is recommended	Grade 2C
ACCP, American College of Chest Physicians; OAC, oral anticoagulant; INR, international normalized ratio	

Table 5: Recommendations for oral anticoagulation in patients with endocarditis[15]	
Patients subgroup	**ACCP grading recommendation**
In patients with a mechanical prosthetic valve and endocarditis who have no contraindications, continuation of long-term vitamin K antagonist is recommended	Grade 2C
ACCP, American College of Chest Physicians	

Warfarin versus Acenocoumarol in Valvular Heart Disease Management

In VHD patients requiring therapy with VKAs, the stability of oral anticoagulation therapy is crucial in preventing thromboembolic as well as bleeding complications.[16]

The anticoagulation strategy with bioprosthetic valves postoperative event registry (ANSWER) study results indicated that about 20% of patients receiving bioprosthetic valve replacement failed to reach therapeutic levels with warfarin treatment. Further, the study results showed that patients who were treated with warfarin had similar rates of embolic events compared to those who were not treated with warfarin (2.8% vs. 3.1%, $p = 0.884$). A substantially higher incidence of bleeding was seen with warfarin compared to no warfarin treatment (12% vs. 3%, $p = 0.0012$). After achievement of an initial therapeutic INR during the 6-month follow-up period, at least one subsequent subtherapeutic INR (<2.0) was observed in 78% of patients and at least one supratherapeutic INR (>3.0) was observed in 57% of patients.[17]

In an observational, comparative, 1-year clinical study, acenocoumarol was found to have significantly better anticoagulation stability with therapeutic INR values covering a longer treatment duration compared to warfarin, though both drugs produced similar quality of individual anticoagulation control in patients with non-valvular AF.[18]

Low-intensity Anticoagulation with Acenocoumarol for Patients with Valvular Heart Disease

A retrospective, nonrandomized study that evaluated the combined use of aspirin and moderate-intensity oral anticoagulant in patients who under-

Table 6: Comparison of two levels of anticoagulant therapy[20]

Parameter	Follow-up	Transient ischemic attack	Bleeding complications (%)
Group A (INR 2.0–2.99)	626 months (12.3 months/patient)	1.92/100 patient-years	3.9
Group B (INR 3.0–4.5)	486 months (10.1 months/patient)	4.94/100 patient-years	20.8

INR, international normalized ratio

went valve replacement showed that moderate-intensity anticoagulation was associated with a lesser incidence of thromboembolic complications, even in those receiving first-generation caged-ball prosthetic valves.[19]

In another randomized, blinded study by Altman et al. which compared two levels of anticoagulant therapy with the acenocoumarol–antiplatelet combination in patients with mechanical substitute heart valves, it was observed that an INR of 2-3 was safer than an INR of 3–4.5, as it offered effective protection from thromboembolic events (Table 6).[20]

In an open, randomized, prospective study conducted in an anticoagulation clinic, the effectiveness of a low (target INR = 2) or moderate (target INR = 3) anticoagulation regimen (with acenocoumarol or warfarin) in preventing thromboembolism was assessed in 103 patients with mitral stenosis-associated AF. The study findings showed that low-intensity anticoagulation, as performed in an anticoagulation clinic, was safe and effective in preventing thromboembolic complications, with only one instance of systemic embolism occurring (0.41 per 100 patient/year) in high-risk mitral stenosis patients with associated AF.[21]

LIMITED ROLE OF NEWER ANTICOAGULANTS IN VALVULAR HEART DISEASE

Novel oral anticoagulants (NOACs) belong to the class of either direct thrombin inhibitors or factor Xa inhibitors. These agents have been approved for use in patients with non-valvular AF, to reduce the risk of stroke and systemic embolism. Dabigatran and rivaroxaban are two such Food and Drug Administration (FDA)-approved NOACs.[22] However, they come with certain drawbacks, for instance:

- There are no data currently available indicating the efficacy of lifelong treatment with these agents in patients with prosthetic mechanical valves
- Their use in situations requiring intensive anticoagulation, e.g., patients with recurrent venous thromboembolism or thrombophilic conditions, is not known
- The concept of increasing the dose, causing intensification of anticoagulant efficacy without causing a considerable increase in the risk of bleeding complications with these novel agents, remains unexplored.

Some of the disadvantages of NOACs are listed in box 2.[23]

Recent data state that one arm of the RE-ALIGN trial (aimed to explore the safety of dabigatran in patients with mechanical heart valves) has been

Box 2: Drawbacks of novel oral anticoagulants[23]

Short half-life
- Potential for increased risk of stroke or systemic embolism with poor drug adherence

No routine coagulation monitoring required
- Potential for increased risk of stroke or systemic embolism with poor drug adherence

No coagulation assay easily available to precisely measure anticoagulation effect
- Cannot titrate dose
- Cannot assess cause for failure of therapy (poor adherence vs. failure)
- Cannot easily assess degree of coagulation inhibition in emergent situations such as need for urgent surgery or in the setting of life-threatening bleeding
- No antidote or well-established procedure for reversing anticoagulation in emergent situations

Cost

Box 3: Indications where vitamin K antagonists will likely remain the front-line long term oral anticoagulants[10]

Rheumatic atrial fibrillation

Mechanical prosthetic valves

Subsets of patients with non-valvular atrial fibrillation
- Poor renal function
- Patients with expected poor compliance, in whom monitoring can serve to improve adherence*
- Patients with sufficiently stable INR*
- Patients who will not be able to afford the increased direct costs of the new oral anticoagulants

*Relative contraindications to the use of novel agents.

INR, international normalized ratio

terminated because of the possibly increased occurrence thromboembolic events with one or more dosages of dabigatran used in the study.[24] In addition, NOACs may have a tendency to accumulate in patients with severe renal impairment.[10]

There are several situations in which VKAs, compared to NOACs, may remain first-line agents (Box 3).[10]

GUIDELINE RECOMMENDATIONS FOR ANTICOAGULANT THERAPY IN VALVULAR HEART DISEASE MANAGEMENT

Recommendations for anticoagulant therapy management of VHD as per the ESC are summarized in table 7.[10]

RECOMMENDED INR FOR PROSTHETIC VALVES

Various prosthetic valves are implanted in different positions in the heart, depending on the disease condition. These prosthetic valves can be broadly classified into two types (Box 4).

Table 7: The European Society of Cardiology recommendations for management of valvular heart disease[10]

Patient indication	Recommendation
Patients with rheumatic mitral valve disease complicated by the presence of left atrial thrombus	VKA therapy (target INR, 2.5; range, 2.0–3.0)
Patients with rheumatic mitral valve disease and normal sinus rhythm with a left atrial diameter more than 55 mm	VKA therapy (target INR, 2.5; range, 2.0–3.0)
Patients with rheumatic mitral valve disease complicated by atrial fibrillation, previous systemic embolism, or both	VKA therapy (target INR, 2.5; range, 2.0–3.0)
All patients with a mechanical heart valve	VKA intensity to be regulated as per the: • Thrombogenicity of prosthesis • The position (aortic vs mitral/tricuspid/pulmonary) • Associated thromboembolic risk factors Routine prescription of antiplatelet drugs is not recommended. Routine addition of aspirin to VKA is not recommended in case of coexistent coronary heart disease.
Patients with bioprosthetic valves in the mitral position	VKA therapy for the first 3 months of valve insertion
The addition of antiplatelet agents to anticoagulation must be: • Individualized (balancing risks and benefits), • Restricted to specific indications, and • Combined with only low-intensity anticoagulation (INR ≤3)	
VKA, vitamin K antagonists; INR, international normalized ratio	

Box 4: Types of prosthetic valve[11]

1. Mechanical
   - Caged ball
   - Tilting disc:
     - Single leaflet
     - Bileaflet
2. Bioprosthetic
   - Heterograft
   - Homograft

Different levels of anticoagulation are required based on the position and type of valve. Tables 8 and 9 list the different INR levels required for adequate anticoagulation in patients with prosthetic valves, depending on the valve type, position of the valve, and associated conditions.[25]

Table 8: Recommended INR in mechanical heart valve replacement and bioprosthetic valve replacement[25]

Mechanical heart valve replacement	
Uncomplicated bileaflet aortic Uncomplicated tilting disc aortic	2.0–3.0
Uncomplicated aortic, and atrial fibrillation	2.5–3.5 or 2.0–3.0 + Aspirin (80–100 mg od)
Uncomplicated bileaflet mitral Uncomplicated tilting disc mitral	2.5–3.5
Additional risk factors, systemic embolism, caged ball valve or caged disc valve	2.5–3.5 + Aspirin (80–100 mg od)
Bioprosthetic valve replacement	
Mitral, aortic , atrial fibrillation, left atrial thrombus, permanent pacemaker, systemic embolism	2.0–3.0
Normal sinus rhythm	Long-term Aspirin (80 mg od)

Table 9: Recommended international normalized ratio (INR) in bioprosthetic valve replacement[25]

	International normalized ratio
Mitral	2.0–3.0
Aortic	2.0–3.0
Atrial fibrillation	2.0–3.0
Left atrial thrombus	2.0–3.0
Permanent pacemaker	2.0–3.0
Systemic embolism	2.0-3.0
Normal sinus rhythm	Long-term Aspirin (80 mg od)

KEY POINTS

- The prevalence of RHD accounts for significant morbidity and mortality worldwide, and the prevalence is particularly high in India, accounting for 25–45% of all acquired heart diseases
- Valvular heart disease is frequently complicated by AF, resulting in an increased risk of stroke in such patients
- Vitamin K antagonists remain the anticoagulation therapy of choice in patients with valvular AF and those with prosthetic valves, in the prevention of thromboembolic events
- Acenocoumarol is associated with better INR stability over a longer duration compared to warfarin in AF
- Studies have found low-intensity acenocoumarol therapy to be safe and effective
- Newer anticoagulants are associated with certain drawbacks and are contradicted in RHD and in the presence of mechanical prosthetics
- Guidelines such as those proposed by the ESC provide suggestions for the effective management of antithrombotic therapy in VHD
- Specific INR target values are recommended for prosthetic valves, depending on the position, type, and extent of thrombogenicity exhibited by that specific device.

REFERENCES

1. Mahmood KT, Anees M, Asghar A. Valvular heart diseases-A review. J Biomed Sci Res. 2011;3(1):315-21.
2. Dey I, Das B, Dey S. Valvular heart diseases and its impact: An assessment among patients attending a tertiary hospital in Kolkata. Int J Med Res Health Sci. 2014;3(3):521-5.
3. National Heart Foundation of Australia (NHFA) and the Cardiac Society of Australia and New Zealand (CSANZ) Diagnosis and management of acute rheumatic fever and rheumatic heart disease in Australia—An evidence-based review. (2006). Management of rheumatic heart disease. [online] Available from http://doctor-ru.org/main/1800/1805.pdf. [Accessed February, 2017].
4. Bhandari S, Subramanyam K, Trehan N. Valvular heart disease: Diagnosis and management. JAPI. 2007;55:575-84.
5. Darby AE, DiMarco JP. Management of atrial fibrillation in patients with structural heart disease. Circulation. 2012;125(7):945-57.
6. Grigioni F, Avierinos JF, Ling LH, Scott CG, Bailey KR, Tajik AJ, et al. Atrial fibrillation complicating the course of degenerative mitral regurgitation: determinants and long-term outcome. J Am Coll Cardiol. 2002;40(1):84-92.
7. Wolf PA, Dawber TR, Thomas HE Jr, Kannel WB. Epidemiologic assessment of chronic atrial fibrillation and risk of stroke: the fiamingham study. Neurology. 1978;28(10):973-7.
8. Ahmad S, Wilt H. Stroke prevention in atrial fibrillation and valvular heart disease. Open Cardiovasc Med J. 2016;10:110-6.
9. Coulshed N, Epstein EJ, McKendrick CS, Galloway RW, Walker E. Systemic embolism in mitral valve disease. Br Heart J. 1970;32(1):26-34.
10. De Caterina R, Husted S, Wallentin L, Andreotti F, Arnesen H, Bachmann F, et al. Vitamin K antagonists in heart disease: current status and perspectives (Section III). Position paper of the ESC Working Group on Thrombosis—Task Force on Anticoagulants in Heart Disease. Thromb Haemost. 2013;110(6):1087-107.
11. Whitlock RP, Sun JC, Fremes SE, Rubens FD, Teoh KH; American College of Chest Physicians. Antithrombotic and thrombolytic therapy for valvular disease: Antithrombotic Therapy And Prevention of Thrombosis, 9th ed: American College of Chest Physicians Evidence-Based Clinical Practice Guidelines. Chest. 2012;141(2 Suppl):e576S-600S.
12. Gohlke-Bärwolf C. Anticoagulation in valvar heart disease: new aspects and management during non-cardiac surgery. Heart. 2000;84(5):567-72.
13. Gohlke-Bärwolf C, Kremer R. Prevention of thromboembolic events in valvular heart disease. Acta Cardiologica. 1995;51(2):129-42.
14. Wipf JE. Anticoagulation and atrial fibrillation. Putting the results of clinical trials into practice. West J Med. 1995;163(2):145-52.
15. Salem DN, Stein PD, Al-Ahmad A, Bussey HI, Horstkotte D, Miller N, et al. Antithrombotic therapy in valvular heart disease—native and prosthetic: the Seventh ACCP Conference on Antithrombotic and Thrombolytic Therapy. Chest. 2004;126(3 Suppl):457S-82S.
16. Horstkotte D, Piper C. Management of patients with heart valve diseases in 2008. What has changed in the last three decades? Deutsche Medizinische Wochenschrift. 2008;133:S280-S284.
17. Brennan JM, Alexander KP, Wallace A, Hodges AB, Laschinger JC, Jones KW, et al. Patterns of anticoagulation following bioprosthetic valve implantation: observations from ANSWER. J Heart Valve Dis. 2012;21(1):78-87.
18. Kulo A, Kusturica J, Kapić E, Becić F, Rakanović-Todić M, Burnazović-Ristić L, et al. Better stability of acenocoumarol compared to warfarin treatment in one-year observational, clinical study in patients with nonvalvular atrial fibrillation. Med Glas (Zenica). 2011;8(1):9-14.
19. Albertal J, Sutton M, Pereyra D, Segura EV, Aramburu DF, Lardani H, et al. Experience with moderate intensity anticoagulation and aspirin after mechanical valve replacement. A retrospective, non-randomized study. J Heart Valve Dis. 1993;2(3):302-7.
20. Altman R, Rouvier J, Gurfinkel E, D'Ortencio O, Manzanel R, de La Fuente L, et al. Comparison of two levels of anticoagulant therapy in patients with substitute heart valves. J Thorac Cardiovasc Surg. 199;101(3):427-31.

21. Pengo V, Barbero F, Biasiolo A, Pegoraro C, Noventa F, Iliceto S. Prevention of thromboembolism in patients with mitral stenosis and associated atrial fibrillation: effectiveness of low intensity (INR target 2) oral anticoagulant treatment. Thromb Haemost. 2003;89(4):760-4.
22. Mekaj YH, Mekaj AY, Duci SB, Miftari EI. New oral anticoagulants: their advantages and disadvantages compared with vitamin K antagonists in the prevention and treatment of patients with thromboembolic events. Ther Clin Risk Manag. 2015;11:967-77.
23. Tsiara S, Pappas K, Boutsis D, Laffan M. New oral anticoagulants: should they replace heparins and warfarin? Hellenic J Cardiol. 2011;52(1):52-67.
24. Medscape. (2012). Dabigatran RE-ALIGN phase 2 mechanical-valve trial partly halted. [online] Available from http://www.medscape.com/viewarticle/791351. [Accessed February, 2017].
25. Ramteke G. (2007). Anticoagulation therapy for prosthetic valves. [online] Available from www.apiindia.org/pdf/medicine_update_2007/25.pdf. [Accessed February, 2017].

11

Anticoagulation in Special Situations: Pregnancy

Uday M Jadhav, Yugandhar Bachhu

INTRODUCTION

Thromboembolic diseases are a cause of significant mortality and are a major public health burden. Certain sections of the patient population are at an increased risk of thromboembolic disorders and require anticoagulation therapy. In such situations, there might also be a higher risk of adverse side effects, such as bleeding complications, due to anticoagulant therapy.[1] This chapter focuses on the different aspects of anticoagulation during pregnancy.

ANTICOAGULATION IN PREGNANCY

Indications for Anticoagulation Therapy in Pregnancy

The risk of thromboembolism is particularly high among pregnant women, due to the increased activation of plasma fibrinogen, von Willebrand factor, and factors V, VII, VIII, IX, X, and XII during late pregnancy. Thromboembolism can be dangerous in women at a higher risk of embolism, such as those with valvular heart disease. Additionally, increased estrogen and elastase levels during pregnancy may lead to structural changes in the blood vessel walls and increased fragility. Further, there is an increased risk of deep vein thrombosis (DVT), due to compression of the inferior vena cava that occurs as a result of an enlarging uterus.[2]

During pregnancy, anticoagulation therapy may be indicated:[3]

- As a prophylactic measure against the development of venous and arterial thromboembolic incidence in some high-risk situations
- For the therapeutic management of established arterial or venous thromboembolic complications.

Oral Anticoagulation in Special Situations During Pregnancy

Venous Thromboembolism

Pregnant women are at a sixfold increased risk of DVT incidence compared to nonpregnant women. Approximately 1 in every 100,000 pregnant women succumbs to pulmonary embolism (PE). In developed countries, PE is the leading cause of death in pregnant women.[4] The American College of Chest Physicians (ACCP) recommends anticoagulation therapy with low molecular weight heparin (LMWH) throughout pregnancy, for venous thromboembolism (VTE) prophylaxis. In women with acute VTE, prolonged treatment for at least 6 weeks postpartum is recommended.[5]

Valvular Heart Disease

During pregnancy, the increased risk of adverse maternal and fetal outcomes requires careful management of valvular heart disease conditions.[1]

In pregnant women with mechanical valve prosthesis who are at a lower risk of valve thrombosis, coumarin derivatives are reported to be relatively safer than unfractionated heparin (UFH) and LMWH. Although teratogenic, the risk of embryopathy is probably lower with vitamin K antagonists (VKAs) when used at a dose <5 mg (for warfarin) daily. However, no definite conclusions can be drawn. Similarly, acenocoumarol, at a dose <2.0 mg, may be considered safe in such populations. The risk of embryopathy with coumarin derivatives can be eliminated by substituting coumarin derivatives with UFH or LMWH during the 6th–12th week of pregnancy.[6]

A case study reported that the use of acenocoumarol throughout the second and third trimesters in a pregnant woman with a mechanical heart valve caused no embryopathy in the newborn.[7,8] The use of VKAs such as acenocoumarol is considered to be safe in breastfeeding mothers, as VKAs are not secreted in the milk in an active form.[8]

The therapeutic use of oral anticoagulants is reportedly beneficial in patients with valvular atrial fibrillation who are at a high risk of thromboembolism. Immediate anticoagulation with UFH followed by LMWH in the first and final trimesters and LMWH, or oral anticoagulants in the second trimester, are recommended.[1]

The European Society of Cardiology (ESC) recommendations for the management of valvular heart disease during pregnancy are summarized in table 1.[8]

Table 1: Management of valvular heart disease in pregnancy[8]

Recommendations	Class*	Level**
Mitral stenosis		
In patients with symptoms or pulmonary hypertension, restricted activities and β1-selective blockers are recommended	I	B
Diuretics are recommended when congestive symptoms persist despite β-blockers	I	B
Patients with severe MS should undergo intervention before pregnancy	I	C
Therapeutic anticoagulation is recommended in the case of atrial fibrillation, left atrial thrombosis, or prior embolism	I	C
Percutaneous mitral commissurotomy should be considered in pregnant patients with severe symptoms or systolic pulmonary artery pressure >50 mmHg despite medical therapy	IIa	C
Aortic stenosis		
Patients with severe AS should undergo intervention pre-pregnancy if		
• They are symptomatic	I	B
• Or LV dysfunction (LVEF <50%) is present	I	C
Asymptomatic patients with severe AS should undergo intervention pre-pregnancy when they develop symptoms during exercise testing	IIa	C

Continued

Continued

Table 1: Management of valvular heart disease in pregnancy[8]		
Recommendations	**Class***	**Level****
Regurgitant lesions		
Patients with severe aortic or mitral regurgitation and symptoms or impaired ventricular function or ventricular dilatation should be treated surgically pre-pregnancy	I	C
Medical therapy is recommended in pregnant women with regurgitant lesions when symptoms occur	I	C
Mechanical valves		
OACs are recommended during the second and third trimesters until the 36th week	I	C
Change of anticoagulation regimen during pregnancy should be implemented in hospital	I	C
If delivery starts while on OACs, cesarean delivery is indicated	I	C
OAC should be discontinued and dose-adjusted UFH (a PTT >2 × control) or adjusted-dose LMWH (target anti-Xa level 4–6 h planned delivery and restarted 4–6 h after delivery if there is no bleeding complications)	I	C
Immediate echocardiography is indicated in women with mechanical valves presenting with dyspnea and/or an embolic event.	I	C
Continuation of OACs should be considered during the first trimester if the warfarin dose required for therapeutic anti-coagulation is <5 mg/day (or phenprocoumon <3 mg/day or acenocoumarol <2 mg/day), after patient information and consent.	IIa	C
Discontinuation of OAC between weeks 6 and 12 and replacement by adjusted-dose UFH (a PTT ≥2 × control; in high risk patients applied as intravenous infusion) or LMWH twice daily (with dose adjustment according to weight and target anti-Xa level 4–6 h post-dose 0.8–1.2 U/mL) should be considered in patients with a warfarin dose required of >5 mg/day (or phenprocoumon >3 mg/day or acenocoumarol >2mg/day).	IIb	C
Discontinuation of OACs between weeks 6 and 12 and replacement by UFH or LMWH under strict dose control (as described above) may be considered on an individual basis in patients with warfarin dose required for therapeutic anticoagulation <5 mg/day (or phenprocoumon <3 mg/day or acenocoumarol <2 mg/day).	IIb	C
Continuation of OACs may be considered between weeks 6 and 12 in patients with a warfarin dose required for therapeutic anticoagulation >5 mg/day (or phenprocoumon >3 mg/day or acenocoumarol >2 mg/day).	IIb	C
LMWH should be avoided, unless anti-Xa levels are monitored.	III	C

aPTT, activated partial thromboplastin time; AS, aortic stenosis; LMWH, low molecular weight heparin; LVEF, left ventricular ejection fraction; MS, mitral stenosis; OACs, oral anticoagulants; UFH, unfractionated heparin.

*Class of recommendation.

**Level of evidence.

Since new oral anticoagulants (Pregnancy Category C-dabigatran, Category C-rivaroxaban, Category B-apixaban) are not backed up by sufficient well-controlled studies in the pregnant population, their use must involve the careful assessment of potential benefits and possible risks.[1]

KEY POINTS

- Thromboembolism is a major risk factor in pregnant women, due to the increase in coagulation factors
- Anticoagulation is indicated in the treatment of pregnant women at increased risk of venous and arterial thromboembolism
- Oral anticoagulants have been recommended for the management of valvular heart disease and venous thromboembolism in pregnant women.

REFERENCES

1. Oral anticoagulation in special population and conditions. JAPI. 2014;62(6):34-42.
2. Toyoda K. Antithrombotic therapy for pregnant women. Neurol Med Chir. 2013; 53(8):526-30.
3. Robin F, Lecuru F, Desfeux P, Boucaya V, Taurelle R. Anticoagulant therapy in pregnancy. Eur J Obstet Gynecol Reprod Biol. 1999;83(2):171-7.
4. Michota F, Merli G. Anticoagulation in special patient populations. Cleve Clin J Med.2005;72:37-42.
5. Bates SM, Greer IA, Middeldorp S, Veenstra DL, Prabulos AM, Vandvik PO, et al. VTE, thrombophilia, antithrombotic therapy, and pregnancy: Antithrombotic Therapy and Prevention of Thrombosis, 9th ed: American College of Chest Physicians Evidence-Based Clinical Practice Guidelines. Chest. 2012;141(2 Suppl):e691S-736S.
6. Pieper P, Balci A, Van Dijk A. Pregnancy in women with prosthetic heart valves. Neth Heart J. 2008;16(12):406-11.
7. Stefanidis K, Papoutsis D, Daskalakis G, Loutradis D, Antsaklis A. Acenocoumarol and pregnancy outcome in a patient with mitral valve prosthesis: a case report. Fetal Diagn Ther. 2009;25(1):115-8.
8. European Society of Gynecology (ESG); Association for European Paediatric Cardiology (AEPC); German Society for Gender Medicine (DGesGM), Regitz-Zagrosek V, Blomstrom Lundqvist C, Borghi C, et al. ESC Guidelines on the management of cardiovascular diseases during pregnancy: the Task Force on the Management of Cardiovascular Diseases during Pregnancy of the European Society of Cardiology (ESC). Eur Heart J. 2011;32(24):3147-97.

12

Anticoagulation in Special Populations: Geriatric and Pediatric

Deependra Bhatnagar

INTRODUCTION

Thromboembolic diseases are a cause of significant mortality and are a major public health burden. Certain sections of the population are at an increased risk of thromboembolic disorders and require anticoagulation therapy. There might also be a higher risk of adverse side effects, such as bleeding complications, due to anticoagulant therapy in such population.[1] This chapter focuses on different aspects of anticoagulation in two such populations, viz. the geriatric and pediatric populations.

ANTICOAGULATION IN GERIATRIC POPULATION

Factors Affecting Use of Anticoagulants in the Elderly

The elderly population is at an increased risk of thromboembolism and hemorrhage. Atrial fibrillation is the most common cardiac condition encountered among the elderly. Although heparin congeners have been proven to be effective anticoagulant agents in this population, VKAs remain the mainstay of long-term anticoagulation therapy. However, there are certain factors that may affect the use of anticoagulants in the elderly; these include:[1]

Risk of Hemorrhage

The intensity of anticoagulation, as well intrinsic patient characteristics, contributes largely to bleeding risk. It has been observed that an international normalized ratio (INR) of more than 3.0 is associated with a higher risk of bleeding than that maintained in the range of 2.0 and 3.0. Hence, careful control and monitoring of INR will result in safer anticoagulation therapy with reduced bleeding complications.

Reduced Renal Function

A reduction in renal function has been associated with an increase in age. Since heparin congeners and certain direct coagulation factor inhibitors such as fondaparinux, dabigatran, and rivaroxaban are largely eliminated in the urine, there might be an increased possibility of accumulation of these drugs. Therefore, careful assessment is required prior to their prescription in the elderly.

Comorbid Conditions

Certain comorbid conditions in the elderly may predispose them to bleeding complications; these include hypertension, ischemic stroke, cerebrovascular diseases, serious heart conditions, liver disease, diabetes, and alcoholism.

Risk of Fall

Elderly patients having AF are at high risk of falls; this in turn leads to an increased risk of intracranial hemorrhage. A higher rate of AF-associated ischemic stroke is also seen in such patients. Anticoagulation could thus prove beneficial in such cases.

Pharmacological Aspects[2]

The pharmacological aspects that may affect the absorption, distribution, metabolism, and clearance of antithrombotic drugs in the elderly are depicted in figure 1. These age-related factors need to be considered for effective antithrombotic therapy management.

Underutilization of Oral Anticoagulants in Elderly

Elderly patients are associated with a two-three-fold increase in bleeding and intracranial hemorrhage. Physicians are reluctant to prescribe oral anticoagulants to elderly patients who have an increased susceptibility to falls, as this corresponds to a fourfold increased risk of traumatic intracranial hemorrhage. These factors may explain the significant underutilization of vitamin K antagonists (VKAs) in the geriatric population.[2]

Even though aged individuals have characteristics that might place them at an elevated risk of bleeding, they also possess factors that make them more likely to benefit from antithrombotic therapy.[3] Incidentally, in the BAFTA (Birmingham Atrial Fibrillation Treatment of the Aged) trial,

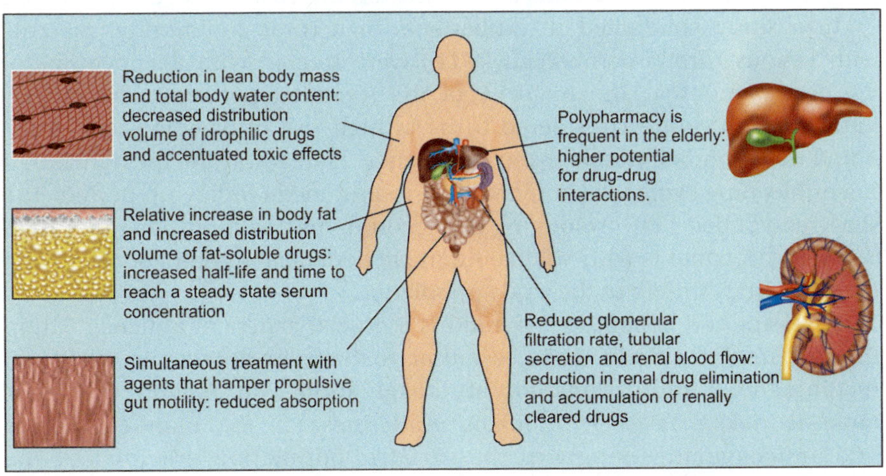

Fig. 1: Age-related pharmacokinetic changes affecting antithrombotic drug therapy[2]

a randomized comparison of warfarin versus aspirin in 973 patients with atrial fibrillation, aged 75 years, the yearly risk of the combined primary endpoint of stroke, intracranial hemorrhage, or clinically significant embolism was 1.8% in patients who received warfarin and 3.8% in those who received aspirin [relative risk: 0.48, 95% confidence interval (CI): 0.28–0.80, p = 0.003]. The study supports the use of anticoagulation therapy in patients aged over 75 years.[4]

Since VKAs are underutilized in the elderly, who face the highest ischemic risk, it is imperative to develop strategies that minimize bleeding risk in this population; these include:[3]

- Blood pressure control
- Interventions to reduce falls
- Careful and vigilant monitoring of INR
- Prevention of excessive anticoagulation
- Making use of predictive tools.

Choosing Anticoagulants for the Elderly Population

Certain factors should be taken into consideration while selecting anticoagulants for the elderly, such as the degree of renal impairment. Vitamin K antagonists are primarily metabolized in the liver, unlike other anticoagulants, which largely depend on renal excretion. This renders VKAs more beneficial in patients with renal impairment, as they do not require dose adjustments. However, novel anticoagulants such as dabigatran depend mainly on renal excretion; since renal impairment is common among the elderly, there might be an accumulation of the anticoagulant and subsequent over-coagulation. Hence, dose adjustments are necessary during therapy in such cases.[1]

Another aspect to be considered is that elderly patients who present with atrial fibrillation are often prescribed antiplatelet agents in combination with anticoagulants; this leads to a significant increase in bleeding risk.[1]

In a study conducted in outpatients in a rural community, patients with venous thromboembolism (VTE) were treated with acenocoumarol for over 6 months. The majority of the included patients were elderly individuals, who are considered to be at high risk of bleeding. The study noted no thromboembolic event recurrence or death. A 3% incidence of a major bleeding event was noted in a 13-month mean follow-up period. The study concluded that prolonging acenocoumarol treatment for more than 6 months in patients with VTE could prove beneficial in outpatients having characteristics similar to the study population.[5]

Assessing the benefit-to-risk ratio is a crucial aspect of anticoagulation therapy in the elderly. It is essential to have in-depth knowledge of recommended indications for anticoagulation and related thromboembolic risks.[3] Table 1 indicates guidelines for the management of oral anticoagulant therapy in the geriatric population provided by the American Geriatric Society (AGS).[6]

Table 1: Management of oral anticoagulation in the elderly[6]

<table>
<tr><td>Initiation of therapy</td><td colspan="2">• Obtain baseline INR (and APTT if on heparin)
• Determine if drug interactions with warfarin are present
• Initial dosage should be an estimate of the average daily dosage of warfarin, usually less than 5 mg daily in the elderly due to increased pharmacodynamic activity
• Discontinue heparin, if being administered concurrently, after the INR has been in the therapeutic range for at least two measurements taken ≥24 hours apart</td></tr>
<tr><td>Monitoring of therapy</td><td colspan="2">• Monitor INR daily until stable; a therapeutic INR is usually achieved in 5–7 days
• The INR can be monitored 2–3 times weekly for 1–2 weeks, then weekly for one month, and monthly thereafter. More frequent monitoring is required in some patients, particularly during changes in medications, particularly antibiotics, and changes in diet</td></tr>
<tr><td rowspan="4">Managing high INR values</td><td>INR 3.0–5.0
No significant bleeding</td><td>• Withhold one dose or lower the dose
• Resume therapy when INR in desired range</td></tr>
<tr><td>INR 5.0–9.0
No significant bleeding</td><td>• Withhold 1–2 doses, resume when INR in desired range
• Consider vitamin K1 (1–2.5 mg p.o.), especially if increased bleeding risk
• If urgent correction required, give vitamin K1 (2–4 mg p.o.); if INR remains high give additional Vitamin K1 (1–2 mg p.o.)
Grade 2C evidence as compared with no treatment</td></tr>
<tr><td>INR >9.0
No significant bleeding</td><td>• Withhold warfarin; give vitamin K1 (3–5 mg p.o.)
• Closely monitor INR; if not substantially reduced in 24–48 h, may require additional vitamin K1</td></tr>
<tr><td>Significant bleeding</td><td>• Discontinue warfarin
• Administer vitamin K1 (10 mg slow IV infusion); supplemented with fresh plasma or prothrombin complex concentrate, depending on urgency; vitamin K1 injections can be repeated every 12 h. (grade 2C)</td></tr>
<tr><td>Managing oral anti-coagulation during invasive procedures</td><td>Low risk for thrombo-embolism
• No VTE >3 mos.
• AF without history of stroke</td><td>• Stop warfarin about 4 days prior to procedure
• Consider short term LMWH or LDUH when INR is reduced if procedure increases risk for thrombosis</td></tr>
</table>

Continued

Continued

Table 1: Management of oral anticoagulation in the elderly[6]

	• Bileaflet mechanical valve in the aortic position	• Resume warfarin following
	• Intermediate risk for thromboembolism	• Stop warfarin about 4 days prior to procedure and allow INR to return to normal range • Administer LMWH or LDUH (5000 IU SC) about 2 days prior to procedure; and following the procedure • Resume warfarin and discontinue LDUH when INR is therapeutic for ≥48 h
	High risk for thromboembolism • VTE in <3 months • History of VTE • Mechanical cardiac valve in mitral position • Old model cardiac valve (ball/cage)	• Stop warfarin about 4 days prior to procedure and allow INR to fall to normal range • Administer full dose heparin (SC or IV) as INR falls, and discontinue about 5 hours prior to procedure; or alternately administer LMWH until 12–24 h prior to the procedure • Resume heparin or LMWH and warfarin after procedure and discontinue LDUH when INR is therapeutic for ≥48 h

INR, international normalized ratio; APTT, activated partial thromboplastin time; VTE, venous thromboembolism; LMWH, low molecular weight heparin; LDUH, low-dose unfractionated heparin

ANTICOAGULATION IN CHILDREN

Issues Affecting Anticoagulation in Children

Over the past decade, there has been an increase in the incidence of VTE in children. Children differ from adults in the underlying pathology of thromboembolism and also in the response to therapy. The pediatric population may also require more frequent monitoring of therapy compared to the adult population.[7]

The issues that should be considered while prescribing anticoagulant therapy in children include:[7]

- The epidemiology of thromboembolism in the pediatric population differs from that in the adult population
- The hemostatic cascade in children is a dynamic, evolving process affecting the frequency and natural history of thromboembolism, as well as response to therapeutic agents

- Certain pharmacokinetic parameters such as distribution, binding, half-life, and clearance are age-dependent
- The frequency, severity, and type of illnesses vary with age
- The nature of co-medication varies with age
- The effective delivery of some therapies is hindered due to limited vascular access; the choice becomes limited, as some drugs are introduced through the parenteral route
- Diet also influences the choice of anticoagulant
- Compliance is difficult to monitor in infants who may not cooperate.

Vitamin K Antagonists in Children

Vitamin K antagonists used in the thrombolytic prophylaxis of children possess several limitations, such as:[7]

- Need for frequent monitoring
- Presence of vitamin K in infant formula
- Dosage available solely in the form of tablets in some countries
- Drug and food interactions.

Acenocoumarol is the preferred anticoagulant in some European and South American countries. Table 2 provides the pediatric dosage, INR range and monitoring frequency of VKAs.

Woods A et al. reported the long-term experience of acenocoumarol plus aspirin in 31 children (5 months to 16 years) with cardiac valve replacement (mitral n = 20; aortic and mitral-aortic n = 4 each; tricuspid n = 3) followed up for 1,336 months. With adequate anticoagulation, embolism was seen in 0.74/1,000 patient-months. Close to 94% of patients did not have thromboembolism up to 96 months of follow-up. The incidence of minor and major hemorrhage was 1.49/1,000 and 0.74/1,000 patient-months respectively. The study reported no major difficulty in anticoagulant management with acenocoumarol in children.[8]

An ideal anticoagulant that can improve the pediatric quality of life should offer a simplified treatment regimen, reduced bleeding, rapid onset of action, predictable pharmacokinetic profile, less frequent monitoring, and minimal food or drug interactions.[7]

<table>
<tr><th colspan="3">Table 2: Starting dose, international normalized ratio range, and monitoring frequency of VKAs[7]</th></tr>
<tr><td>In infants</td><td>0.33 mg/kg</td><td rowspan="2">Maintenance of INR at 2.0–3.0, except in prosthetic mechanical heart valves and recurrent thrombotic episodes, where the target INR is 2.5–3.5</td></tr>
<tr><td>In adolescents</td><td>0.09 mg/kg</td></tr>
<tr><td colspan="3">Monitoring frequency
• 1 or 4 times/month, depending on age, change in dose, concurrent administration of other drugs, and patient compliance</td></tr>
</table>

KEY POINTS

- Geriatric Population
    - The elderly are at an increased risk for thromboembolic complications, especially when atrial fibrillation is indicated
    - Vitamin K antagonists are the mainstay of long-term anticoagulant therapy in the elderly
    - Factors such as comorbid conditions, renal function, risk of fall, and hemorrhage, as well as pharmacological aspects, may influence anticoagulant use in the elderly
    - As the elderly have a two-three-fold increased risk of bleeding and intracranial hemorrhage, oral anticoagulation is often underprescribed in this population
    - The development of strategies to minimize the risk of bleeding is important to maximizing the benefits of anticoagulation
    - Careful assessment of the benefit-to-risk ratio is essential for effective anticoagulation therapy in the geriatric population.
- Pediatric Population
    - Children differ from adults in the underlying pathology of thromboembolism, as well as the response to therapy
    - There has been an increase in the incidence of VTE among children in the past decade
    - Vitamin K antagonists therapy requires more frequent monitoring in children than adults.

REFERENCES

1. Oral anticoagulation in special population and condition. JAPI. 2014;62(6):34-42.
2. Capodanno D, Angiolillo DJ. Antithrombotic therapy in the elderly. J Am Coll Card. 2010;56(21):1683-92.
3. Robert-Ebadi H, Le Gal G, Righini M. Use of anticoagulants in elderly patients: practical recommendations. Clin Interv Aging. 2009;4:165-77.
4. Mant J, Hobbs F, Fletcher K, Roalfe A, Fitzmaurice D, Lip GY, et al. Warfarin versus aspirin for stroke prevention in an elderly community population with atrial fibrillation (the Birmingham Atrial Fibrillation Treatment of the Aged Study, BAFTA): a randomised controlled trial. Lancet. 2007;370(9586):493-503.
5. Calvo-Romero JM. Prolonged acenocoumarol treatment in patients with venous thromboembolic disease from a rural area. South Med J. 2007;100(7):725.
6. Jacobs LG. (2001). Current guidelines for practice oral anticoagulation for older adults. Clinical Practice Committee of the American Geriatrics Society. Available from http://www.sigg.it/public/doc/DASCARICARE/155.pdf. [Accessed February, 2017].
7. Dabbous MK, Sakr FR, Malaeb DN. Anticoagulant therapy in pediatrics. J Basic Clin Pharma. 2014;5(2):27-33.
8. Woods A, Vargas J, Berri G, Kreutzer G, Meschengieser S, Lazzari MA. Antithrombotic therapy in children and adolescents. Thrombo Res. 1986;42(3):289-301.

13

Anticoagulation in Special Situations: Cancer

Nitin S Patki

INTRODUCTION

Thromboembolic diseases are a cause of significant mortality and are a considerable public health burden. Certain sections of the population are at an increased risk for thromboembolic disorders and require anticoagulation therapy. Approximately 15% of all cancer patients have been reported to have clinically manifested VTE.[1] This chapter focuses on different aspects of cancer-associated thromboembolism and its management through anticoagulation therapy.

THROMBOEMBOLISM IN CANCER

The relationship between thrombosis and malignancy has been well established for more than 100 years. A dynamic interaction between the cancer cells, host cells, and the coagulation system contributes to the pathogenesis of hypercoagulability in cancer. Tumor cells express a procoagulant molecule involved in the continuous activation of coagulation and increased production of thrombin known as the tissue factor (TF). The upregulation of TF leads to the production of proangiogenic cytokine vascular endothelial growth factor (VEGF), resulting in increased vascular permeability. This allows for an incremental exposure to coagulation factors and a subsequent intensification of the procoagulant environment.[2]

Malignancy is a major predisposing factor for the development of venous thromboembolism (VTE) and pulmonary embolism (PE). Venous thromboembolism constitutes the second most common cause of death after cancer itself. The probability of developing VTE varies among cancer patients and is dependent on factors such as the type of cancer, clinical setting, comorbid conditions, and therapeutic procedures involved. Compared to noncancer patients, oncology patients have been associated with a significantly higher risk of new and recurrent VTE. There is fivefold increased risk of VTE in cancer patients undergoing surgery and a sixfold increased risk in those receiving chemotherapy.[2]

Issues such as long periods of ambulation, difficulty in maintenance of anticoagulation therapy, and poor prognosis warrant intense anticoagulation monitoring in patients with cancer.[1]

VITAMIN K ANTAGONISTS IN CANCER THERAPY: CLINICAL STUDIES

Anticoagulation may be beneficial in the treatment of underlying malignancy. Thrombin and fibrin aid in the adhesion and implantation of tumor cells, and fibrin deposits around tumors may offer protection against immune surveillance. The antifibrin and antithrombin effects of anticoagulant agents may inhibit adhesion as well as helping in the immune clearance of cancer cells.[3]

> Approximately 15% of all cancer patients have been reported to have clinically manifested VTE.

A population-based observational cohort study was conducted to investigate the impact of long-term vitamin K antagonists (VKA) use on the development of newly diagnosed malignancies and on cancer-related overall mortality. The study included 89,787 individuals; VKA exposure was assessed on the basis of anatomical therapeutic chemical (ATC) codes on the drug prescription. It was noted that the patients in the VKA-exposed group were significantly older (76.4 ± 6.8 years vs. 74.8 ± 7.2 years) and followed up for a longer duration compared to the control group (9.1 ± 2.4 years vs. 8.8 ± 2.6 years). After adjustment for age and sex, it was noted that patients exposed to VKA had a lower incidence of cancer (hazard ratio 0.88, $p < 0.015$). Further, the incidence of prostate cancer was significantly reduced (hazard ratio 0.69, $p = 0.008$) among the specific tumors.[4]

The study results support the hypothesis that long-term treatment with VKAs has a protective effect on the development of cancer, especially prostate cancer, in elderly patients. The mechanism of this anticancer effect is suggested to involve thrombin in relation to protease-activated receptors Gas6 and Axl. This Gas6/Axl axis is believed to regulate the invasion, proliferation, and survival of prostate cancer. Since the findings showed a reduced risk of cancer after years of VKA exposure, it has been suggested that the protective effect of VKAs may be exhibited at the stage of tumor initiation or promotion, rather than on an established tumor.[4]

A prospective randomized trial investigated the effect of anticoagulant use as an adjunct to cytotoxic chemotherapy in patients with small-cell lung cancer. The patients were randomized to receive either warfarin or no anticoagulant therapy. Patients with either extensive- or limited-stage cancer were enrolled for the study. The prothrombin time of adjusted-dose warfarin was twice that of the control. There was a statistically significant prolongation of survival demonstrated for patients who received warfarin (median survival 49.5 weeks) compared with those who did not (median survival 23.0 weeks).[5]

Another study conducted in cancer patients analyzed the efficacy and safety of early and short-term thromboprophylaxis with acenocoumarol and dalteparin in the prevention of nonocclusive and occlusive central vein catheter-related thrombosis (CVCRT). The study reported that acenocoumarol was better than dalteparin in the prevention of CVCRT [odds ratio (OR) 0.4, $p = 0.01$].[6]

RECOMMENDATION FOR ANTICOAGULANT TREATMENT IN PATIENTS WITH CANCER[1]

Initiation of therapy with low molecular weight heparin (LMWH) and continuation of therapy for 3–6 months, followed by either LMWH or VKA treatment for an indefinite duration or until the cancer is treated.

KEY POINTS

- There is a well-established relationship between thrombosis and malignancy
- The development of VTE is a major complication in cancer patients
- Long-term VKA therapy has been shown to be beneficial in reducing the incidence of prostate cancer in elderly patients
- An improved rate or survival is associated with VKA therapy in patients with small-cell lung cancer.

REFERENCES

1. Oral anticoagulation in special population and condition. JAPI. 2014;62(6):34-42.
2. Barbosa M. What is the best treatment for a cancer patient with thrombosis? Clin Med Insights Oncol. 2014;8:49-55.
3. Letai A, Kuter DJ. Cancer, coagulation, and anticoagulation. Oncologist. 1999;4(6):443-9.
4. Pengo V, Noventa F, Denas G, Pengo MF, Gallo U, Grion AM, et al. Long-term use of vitamin K antagonists and incidence of cancer: a population-based study. Blood. 2011;117(5):1707-9.
5. Zacharski LR, Henderson WG, Rickles FR, Forman WB, Cornell CJ Jr, Forcier RJ, et al. Effect of warfarin anticoagulation on survival in carcinoma of the lung, colon, head and neck, and prostate. Final report of VA Cooperative Study # 75. Cancer. 1984;53(10):2046-52.
6. De Cicco M, Matovic M, Balestreri L, Steffan A, Pacenzia R, Malafronte M, et al. Early and short-term acenocumarine or dalteparin for the prevention of central vein catheter-related thrombosis in cancer patients: a randomized controlled study based on serial venographies. Ann Oncol. 2009;20(12):1936-42.

14

Anticoagulation in Special Situations: Chronic Kidney Disease

Uday M Jadhav

INTRODUCTION

Thromboembolic diseases are a cause of significant mortality and are a considerable public health burden. Certain sections of the population are at an increased risk of thromboembolic disorders and require anticoagulation therapy.[1] However, an increased risk of therapy-associated bleeding complications is also seen in such patient populations. This chapter focuses on different aspects of chronic kidney disease (CKD)-associated thromboembolism and its management through anticoagulation therapy.

RISK OF THROMBOEMBOLISM IN CHRONIC KIDNEY DISEASE

Chronic kidney disease is a pandemic public health problem. The increasing burden of CKD may be attributed to the increase in the size of aging population and the increase in the prevalence of diabetes mellitus. Several epidemiological studies have shown that patients with all stages of CKD experience higher rates of atherothrombotic diseases and processes with thromboembolic potential [such as atrial fibrillation (AF)] than the general population. This indicates the importance of antithrombotic treatment in such patients. However, as much as they stand to benefit from the use of antithrombotic drugs, CKD patients are also at an increased risk of bleeding complications. Thus, a careful balance of benefits and risks should be maintained.[2]

Factors that may contribute to the prothrombic nature of CKD include:[3]

- Development of prothrombic changes in the vascular endothelium
- Increase in coagulation factors such as fibrinogen, factor VIII, and von Willebrand factor due to CKD-associated chronic inflammation
- Inhibition of clot breakdown due to increased levels of antifibrinolytic proteins such as plasminogen activator inhibitor
- Hyperlipidemia leading to increased risk of cardiovascular thrombosis
- Hemoconcentration and proaggregatory changes in the platelet membrane.

The bleeding risk in CKD may be attributed to anemia-related platelet dysfunction, which can impact the interaction between platelets with the vessel wall.

ANTICOAGULATION IN PATIENTS WITH CHRONIC KIDNEY DISEASE

Prophylaxis with anticoagulant therapy is beneficial in patients with CKD who are at an increased risk of thrombotic situations.[3] The risk of AF is reportedly higher in patients with CKD. The use of vitamin K antagonists (VKAs) has been shown to reduce ischemic complications in patients with mild-to-moderate CKD and AF without significant risk of bleeding.[1] However, CKD may affect the pharmacokinetic characteristics of these antithrombotic drugs in different ways (Box 1). In addition, a 50% reduction in renal excretion may lead to drug accumulation in almost two-thirds of CKD patients.[2]

Vitamin K antagonists are metabolized in the liver; hence, no dosage adjustments are required in patients with CKD, although careful monitoring of the therapy is essential. On the contrary, dosing adjustments are required with heparin congeners and newer anticoagulants, as their elimination is solely through the kidneys, which in turn may result in drug accumulation and over-anticoagulation in patients with renal impairment.[1] In addition, no antidote currently exists to reverse active bleeding caused by newer anticoagulants; also, some newer drugs may be associated with a prolonged therapeutic half-life in patients with CKD stages 4 or 5.[3] The pharmacokinetics of some newer anticoagulants is depicted in figure 1.[2]

Box 1: Pharmacokinetic properties of antithrombotic drugs affected by chronic kidney disease[2]

- Increased bioavailability
- Increased distribution
- Prolonged time to reach maximum drug concentration
- Prolonged half-life
- Reduced excretion

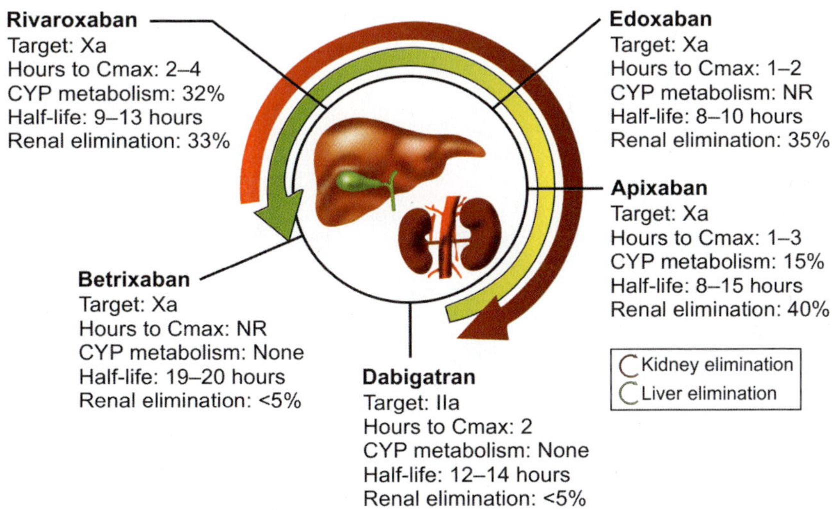

Fig. 1: Pharmacokinetic properties or newer oral anticoagulants[2]

The dosing adjustments and risk of over-coagulation associated with newer anticoagulants, along with the need to assess renal function before their administration, make VKAs a more convenient therapeutic option for patients with CKD.[1]

KEY POINTS

- Patients with CKD have an increased risk of thromboembolic incidence compared to the general population
- Patients with CKD are prothrombic as well as having hemorrhagic tendencies, making antithrombotic therapy either beneficial or harmful in this population
- Newer anticoagulants largely depend on renal excretion and may require dosing adjustments
- A 50% reduction in renal elimination may lead to an accumulation of antithrombotic drugs
- Vitamin K antagonists help reduce ischemic complications in patients with mild-to-moderate CKD who are at an increased risk for AF
- Vitamin K antagonists may be a better treatment option in CKD patients, due to the risk of accumulation and subsequent over-coagulation associated with newer anticoagulants.

REFERENCES

1. Oral anticoagulation in special population and condition. JAPI. 2014;62(6):34-42.
2. Capodanno D, Angiolillo D. Antithrombotic therapy in patients with chronic kidney disease. Circulation. 2012;125(21):2649-61.
3. Hughes S, Szeki I, Nash MJ, Thachil J. Anticoagulation in chronic kidney disease patients—the practical aspects. Clin Kidney J. 2014;7(5):442-9.

15

Anticoagulation in Major and Minor Surgeries

Prashant Vaijyanath

MANAGING ANTICOAGULATION IN PATIENTS UNDERGOING SURGERY

Oral anticoagulants (OACs) are frequently administered in order to avert complications such as thromboembolism in patients with prosthetic heart valves, congestive heart failure, and valvular defects. However, OACs are also associated with a prolonged bleeding time following surgery, because their anticoagulation action is antagonistic to vitamin K, which is necessary for attaining hemostasis.[1]

The international normalized ratio (INR) is used to monitor the anticoagulation level in such patients. For general indications, the recommended therapeutic range of INR is 2–3. However, in patients with prosthetic valves, the recommended INR range is 3–4, in order to maintain strict anticoagulation.[1]

Major general surgery is not recommended in circumstances wherein the INR range is between 2 and 4, due to the possibility of severe hemorrhage, which cannot be controlled without changing or stopping OAC. In case a major surgery is performed without any consideration of changing or discontinuing anticoagulants, there is a serious possibility of severe postoperative bleeding, which could be life-threatening. On the other hand, in minor surgeries, the necessity of changing or discontinuing OAC continues to be unclear.[1]

RISK ASSESSMENT

Risk of Thromboembolism with Discontinuation of Oral Anticoagulants

The interruption of anticoagulation treatment due to surgical or invasive procedures is a major clinical concern. Discontinuation of anticoagulation in patients undergoing surgery increases the risk of thromboembolic complications.[2] A study demonstrated the occurrence of thromboembolic events in 22% of patients following discontinuation of OAC. Moreover, the mortality due to thromboembolism was reported in 4% of patients. The study concluded that the risk of thromboembolic events increases irrespective of the duration of discontinuation if the patient stops taking OAC.[1]

Risk of Hemorrhage with the Continuation of Oral Anticoagulant

Continuation of anticoagulation in patients undergoing surgery enhances the risk of serious bleeding complications.[2] A systematic review of five randomized controlled trials and 11 controlled trials showed no substantial difference in postoperative hemorrhage between patients who stopped OAC treatment and patients who continued OAC with the recommended INR range of 2–4. Moreover, postoperative bleeding was not associated with INR status.[1] The subset of patients in whom a periprocedural alternative to oral anticoagulation is necessary includes patients with atrial fibrillation, prosthetic heart valves, and hypercoagulable states and those with chronic venous thrombosis undergoing surgery.[2]

Hence, while making a decision regarding an anticoagulation protocol, the timing of surgery, bleeding risk, and thromboembolic risk must be taken into consideration.[3]

BRIDGING ANTICOAGULATION

The purpose of bridging anticoagulation is to decrease the period of anticoagulant interruption and, therefore, thromboembolic risk.[4] Bridging anticoagulation involves the administration of a short-acting anticoagulant consisting of subcutaneous (SC) low molecular weight heparin (LMWH) for 1–12 days around the time of the surgery/procedure, when the anticoagulant effect of warfarin is outside the therapeutic range (Fig 1).[5]

Bridging anticoagulation aims to reduce patients' risk of developing stroke; however, it may also increase patients' risk for developing potentially serious bleeding complications after surgery.[5]

Patients in the moderate risk group, based on $CHADS_2$ score, who are undergoing low-bleeding risk surgery and could benefit from bridging anticoagulation include:[4]

- Patients with mechanical bileaflet aortic valve and additional CHADS stroke risk factors

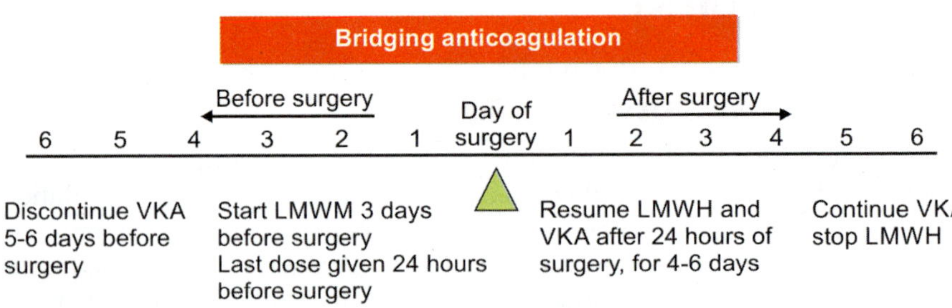

VKA, vitamin K antagonists; LMWH, low molecular weight heparin.

Fig. 1: Bridging anticoagulation[5]

- Patients with AF and a $CHADS_2$ score of 3 or 4, or prior thromboembolism during warfarin interruption
- Patients with venous thromboembolism (VTE) in the past 3–12 months, non-severe thrombophilia, active cancer, and recurrent VTE.

Bridging therapy should not be considered in patients with a moderate risk of bleeding who are undergoing high-bleeding risk procedures such as major cardiac surgery, major orthopedic procedures, carotid endarterectomy, or neurosurgery.[4]

In patients undergoing major surgery, therapeutic-dose LMWH should be delayed for a minimum of 24 hours or longer (48–72 hours) after the operation. Restarting LMWH depends on the clinical evidence of surgical site hemostasis. In an observational study, all patients received LMWH after 12–24 hours of all types of surgery. The study demonstrated a 20% incidence of major bleeding in patients who had major surgery (>1 hour duration), and 0.7% of patients undergoing minor procedures had major bleeding.[4]

PERIOPERATIVE MANAGEMENT OF ANTICOAGULATION

The surgeon should perform a risk assessment of surgery-associated bleeding with or without antithrombotic use and morbidity or mortality related to bleeding. While evaluating the surgical bleeding risk, anesthetic management should also be taken into consideration, particularly in neuraxial regional anesthesia, where the likelihood of bleeding complications is high. Such risk assessment aids in balancing the bleeding risk against the possible morbidity related with the interruption of antiplatelet or anticoagulant treatment.[4]

Evidence suggests that the following surgeries confer a higher bleeding risk in the setting of antithrombotic use:[4]

- Transurethral prostate resection, bladder resection, or tumor ablation
- Pacemaker or implantable defibrillator insertion in which the separation of infraclavicular fascial layers and a lack of suturing of unopposed tissues within the device pocket may predispose to hematoma colonic polyp resection, typically of large (>1–2 cm) polyps, in which bleeding may occur at the transected stalk after hemostatic plug release. Procedures involving highly vascular organs, such as the kidneys, liver, and spleen
- Bowel resection in which bleeding can occur at the anastomotic site
- Major surgery with extensive tissue injuries, such as joint arthroplasty, cancer surgery, and reconstructive plastic surgery
- Cardiac, intracranial, or spinal surgery, especially procedures with small pericardial, intracerebral, or epidural bleeds, can have significant consequences.

The following are some minimally invasive procedures that can be carried out safely even if patients are receiving OAC:[6]

- Ophthalmic surgery
  - Cataract surgery
  - Trabeculectomy
  - Vitreoretinal surgery
- Dental procedures
  - Dental hygiene
  - Simple extractions
  - Restorations
  - Endodontics
  - Prosthetics.

GUIDELINE RECOMMENDATION

The American College of Chest Physicians 2012 guidelines for the perioperative management of VKA therapy are summarized in table 1.[7]

Table 1: American College of Chest Physicians 2012 guidelines: Perioperative management of anticoagulation[7]

Category	Recommendations
In patients who require temporary cession of a VKA prior to surgery	• Discontinue VKAs approximately 5 days before surgery • Restart VKAs approximately 12–24 h after surgery (evening or next morning) and when there is adequate hemostasis
In patients with a mechanical heart valve, atrial fibrillation, or VTE	• Patients at high risk for thromboembolism: Bridging anticoagulation should be considered during cessation of VKA therapy • Patients at low risk for thromboembolism: No bridging anticoagulation during cessation of VKA therapy • Moderate risk of thromboembolism: Judgment should be based on surgery and patient characteristics
In patients who require a minor dental procedure	• Continue VKAs combined with an oral prohemostatic agent or discontinue VKAs 2–3 days before the procedure
In patients who require minor dermatologic procedures	• Continue VKAs around the time of the procedure and optimize local hemostasis
In patients who require cataract surgery	• Continue VKAs around the time of the surgery

VKA, vitamin K antagonists; VTE, venous thromboembolism.

KEY POINTS

- Continuation or discontinuation of OAC in patients undergoing surgery is a dilemma
- Careful planning and evaluation of the risk and benefits are required prior to surgery in patients on OACs
- Bridging anticoagulation refers to the administration of a short-acting anti-coagulant comprising SC low molecular weight heparin (LMWH) for 10–12 days around the time of the surgery/procedure, when the anticoagulant effect of warfarin is outside the therapeutic range
- Bridging anticoagulation can be beneficial in some patients.

REFERENCES

1. Cho YW, Kim E. Is stopping of anticoagulant therapy really required in a minor dental surgery? How about in an endodontic microsurgery? Restor Dent Endod. 2013;38(3):113-8.
2. Jafri SM, Mehta TP. Periprocedural management of anticoagulation in patients on extended warfarin therapy. Semin Thromb Hemost. 2004;30(6):657-64.
3. Thakur NA, Czerwein JK, Butera JN, Palumbo MA. Perioperative management of chronic anticoagulation in orthopaedic surgery. J Am Acad Orthop Surg. 2010;18(12):729-38.
4. McKenzie JL, Douglas G, Bazargan A. Perioperative management of anticoagulation in elective surgery. ANZ J Surg. 2013;83(11):814-20.
5. BRIDGE Study Investigators. Bridging anticoagulation: Is it needed when warfarin is interrupted around the time of a surgery or procedure? Circulation. 2012;125(12):e496-8.
6. Spandorfer J. The management of anticoagulation before and after procedures. Med Clin North Am. 2001;85(5):1109-16.
7. Douketis JD, Spyropoulos AC, Spencer FA, Mayr M, Jaffer AK, Eckman MH, et al. Perioperative management of antithrombotic therapy: Antithrombotic therapy and Prevention of Thrombosis, 9th ed: American College of Chest Physicians Evidence-Based Clinical Practice Guidelines. Chest. 2012;141(2 Suppl):e326S-50S.

16

Anticoagulation in Dental Surgeries

Bhupesh Shah, Deependra Bhatnagar

INTRODUCTION

Continuous anticoagulation therapy has been crucial in preventing thrombo-embolism. However, dental surgery in patients undergoing continuous anticoagulation is widely debated due to the potential risk of hemorrhage.[1] This chapter focuses on various factors influencing dental surgeries in continuously anticoagulated patients.

DENTAL SURGERY IN ANTICOAGULATED PATIENTS

The oral cavity has a rich blood supply and a mucosa that can be bruised, resulting in bleeding. Additionally, proteolytic enzymes in the saliva aid in fibrinolysis and may perpetuate bleeding; however, saliva also aids in thrombin generation through the expression of tissue factor-like substances, thus resulting in a hemostatic environment.[2] Different phases of hemostasis include the following three phases.[3]

Vascular or Vasoconstriction Phase

Vascular damage results in immediate vasoconstriction of damaged blood vessels, preventing excessive blood flow. This lasts about 20 minutes (Fig. 1A).

Platelet Phase

Bleeding is further reduced by the formation of platelet clots formed by the adherence of platelets to the exposed subendothelial collagen (Fig. 1B).

Plasmatic Phase

The sequential activation of coagulation factors leads to the activation of prothrombin and the subsequent formation of the proteolytic enzyme, thrombin. Thrombin mediates the conversion of soluble fibrinogen to insoluble fibrin.

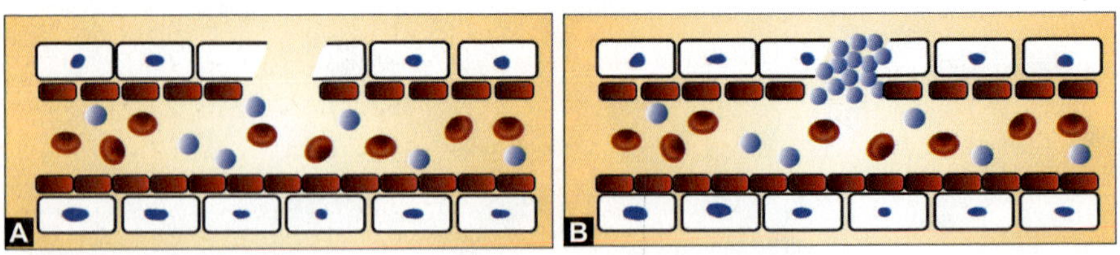

Fig. 1: Phases of hemostasis[3]

Anticoagulant drugs act by blocking the conversion of vitamin K epoxide to its active form by inhibiting the enzyme vitamin K reductase. The formation of coagulation factors dependent on this active form thus gets inhibited, resulting in a subsequent blockage of the coagulation process. This alteration in the hemostatic process may lead to uncontrolled bleeding.[3]

Dental treatment on patients undergoing continuous anticoagulation has therefore been controversial, as physicians need to consider the risk of hemorrhage from the dental procedure as well as risks of thromboembolic events upon withdrawal of anticoagulation treatment.[1]

TYPES OF DENTAL PROCEDURE

Dental procedures taking place in a primary care setting may either be relatively noninvasive, not requiring a prior measurement of international normalized ratio (INR), or potentially invasive and at a higher risk of bleeding. Table 1 provides a list of these procedures.[4]

Risk Assessment: Bleeding versus Thromboembolism

Risk of Bleeding with Continuation of Oral Anticoagulation: Clinical Studies

Several studies have investigated the bleeding risk in patients undergoing oral surgery while under continuous anticoagulation with vitamin K antagonists.

In a prospective study involving patients requiring simple dental extractions, 109 patients were on continuous oral anticoagulation therapy (OAT); another 105 patients were bridged with low molecular weight heparin and had a mean INR of 1.26 + 0.11 on the day of the procedure. Only a few post-interventional minor bleeding events occurred in the two groups. Although the group with permanent anticoagulation had more bleeding incidences, there was no significant difference between the two groups. All minor bleeding complications were easily resolved with local hemostatic measures.[5]

Table 1: Types of dental procedure[4]

Noninvasive procedures	Potentially invasive procedures
Prosthodontics (construction of dentures)	Endodontics (root canal treatment)
Scaling/polishing	Local anesthesia (infiltrations, inferior alveolar nerve block, mandibular blocks)
Conservation work (fillings, crowns, bridges)	• Extractions (single and multiple) • Minor oral surgery • Periodontal surgery • Biopsies • Subgingival scaling

Wahl reviewed 26 papers comprising 2014 dental surgical procedures in 774 patients receiving continuous warfarin therapy, including 1,964 patients undergoing single, multiple, and full-mouth extractions; surgical extractions; alveolectemies; and other surgical procedures. This meta-analysis included patients with an INR of up to 4.0. Although some patients had minor oozing treated with local measures, more than 98% of patients receiving continuous anticoagulants had no serious bleeding problems. Twelve patients (<2%) had postoperative bleeding problems that were not controlled by local measures. Five of these 12 episodes were associated with a supratherapeutic INR.[1] Based on the observations made in this study, it can be concluded that continuation of anticoagulant therapy during dental procedures is not associated with any major complications.

Risk of Discontinuing Oral Anticoagulation: Clinical Study

Perioperative withdrawal of anticoagulation therapy is known to be associated with risk of thromboembolic events. For minor procedures, such as dental surgery, the risk may vary from 0.02% to 1%.[6]

Wahl investigated the impact of discontinuing anticoagulant therapy by reviewing 542 documented cases involving 493 patients in whom anticoagulation therapy was withdrawn specifically for dental procedures. It was reported that 4 patients had serious thromboembolic events leading to death (2 cerebral thromboses, 1 myocardial infarction, and 1 embolus) and one patient had two nonfatal thromboembolic complications (1 cerebral embolus and 1 brachial artery embolus). The incidence of serious thromboembolic complications was observed in 1.0% of patients; 0.9% of cases.[1]

Continuation versus Discontinuation of Anticoagulant Therapy: Comparative Studies

Campbell et al. randomized 25 patients undergoing dentoalveolar surgery to either discontinue warfarin 72–96 hours prior to the surgical intervention or to continue anticoagulants. A further group of individuals not receiving anticoagulants served as controls. No patient in any group had postoperative bleeding sufficiently severe to warrant therapeutic intervention, and there was no significant difference in blood loss between the three groups.[7]

In another study, Sacco et al. randomized 131 patients on OAT to reduced anticoagulation or full anticoagulation. Five hundred and eleven teeth were extracted by the same surgeon. Mild bleeding was observed in 10 cases (15.1%) in the reduced-dosage group, which also required local hemostatic measures to control bleeding. The unmodified-dosage group saw 6 cases (9.2%) of mild bleeding. The difference between the groups was not considered significant. The study concluded that it is not required to reduce OAT in patients undergoing dental extractions, provided local measures of hemostasis are applied.[8]

Evans et al. compared 109 patients undergoing dental extractions who were divided into two groups: (i) control group (warfarin was suspended

Box 1: Local hemostatic measures of controlling bleeding in patients receiving continuous anticoagulation therapy[10]	
• Local Pressure with gauze packs • Gelatin sponge	• Fibrin glue • Tranexamic or e-aminocaproic acid

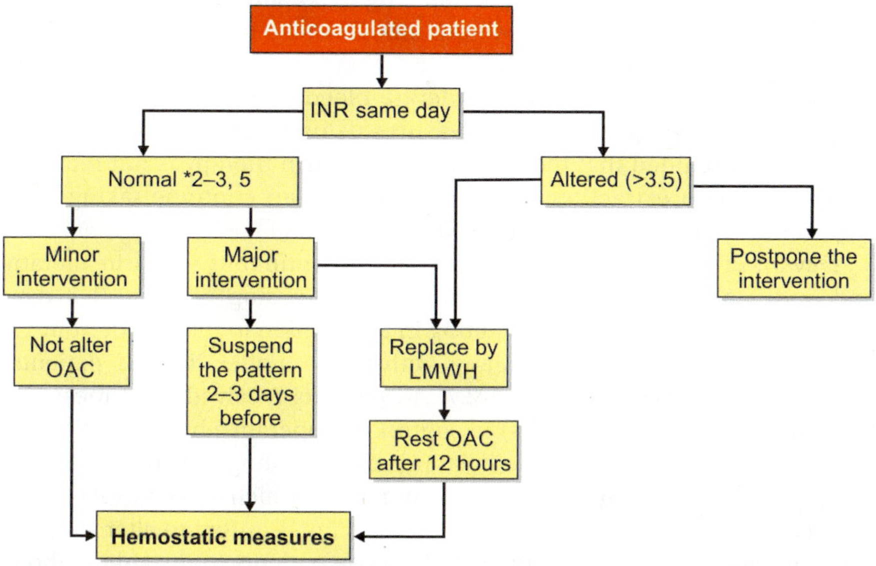

INR, international normalized ratio; OAC, oral anticoagulant; LMWH, low molecular weight heparin.

Fig. 2: Management algorithm for patients with anticoagulation therapy scheduled to undergo invasive dental treatment[3]

two days before the operation; n = 52) and (ii) intervention group (warfarin continued; n = 57). Mild postoperative bleeding was recorded in 15 patients who continued warfarin and in 7 patients in whom warfarin was suspended, the difference being nonsignificant. Bleeding was controlled by patients at home by local hemostatic measures.[9]

The above clinical study supports the notion that it is not required to either withhold or reduce anticoagulation during minor procedures, as local hemostatic measures (Box 1) are able to minimize or control any bleeding events.[10] However, in the case of major elective surgery (over three extractions), when the INR more than 3.5 with coexisting risk factors, it is suggested to suspend anticoagulation 2–3 days before surgery (based on the degree of thromboembolic risk) or to switch to subcutaneous heparin (Fig. 2).[3]

DENTAL EXTRACTION IN PATIENTS ON WARFARIN TREATMENT

Patients undergoing warfarin therapy and intended for surgical procedures may be at a heightened risk of bleeding. Various guidelines exist for the management of such patients prior to surgical intervention. The American

College of Chest Physicians recommends stopping warfarin therapy 5 days before any surgical intervention and also suggests bridging warfarin therapy with low molecular weight heparin. The American Heart Association, however, recommends the reduction of INR to a range 2.0–2.5, along with strict INR monitoring.[11]

A study investigated the risk of bleeding in 35 patients (INR <4) undergoing simple tooth extractions without modifications in their warfarin dose. No significant bleeding was observed following the procedure. Overall, 4 patients (11.4%) experienced moderate bleeding after tooth extraction that could be managed by local measures using local hemostatic agents. The study concluded that modification of warfarin therapy is not required for simple tooth extractions and that patients can continue taking their regular medications, provided the INR is below 3.50.[11]

Devani et al. randomized 65 patients on continuous warfarin therapy and undergoing 133 dental extractions to either stop warfarin 2–3 days prior to surgery (32 patients), resulting in a reduction in mean INR from 2.6 to 1.6, or to continue anticoagulants with no dose alteration (32 patients) and a mean preoperative INR of 2.7. All patients received local measures ("Surgicel" packing and sutures) to control postoperative bleeding. None of the patients had any immediate postoperative bleeding, and only 1 patient from each group had mildly delayed hemorrhage, which was controlled with local measures. The study concluded that it is not required to alter warfarin therapy prior to dental extractions and expose patients to thromboembolic risk; however, INR must be maintained at a therapeutic range of 2.0–4.0, and local measures should be applied to control postoperative bleeding.[12]

IMPACT OF ANTI-INFLAMMATORY DRUGS IN PATIENTS RECEIVING ANTICOAGULATION AND UNDERGOING DENTAL SURGERY

Most dental surgical procedures require postoperative medications such as nonsteroidal anti-inflammatory drugs (NSAIDs), for the management of postoperative pain and inflammation; however, anticoagulants present a contradiction to the use of NSAIDs due to the risk of uncontrolled bleeding resulting from the erosion and ulceration of gastric mucosa. This effect is rarely encountered in low-dose aspirin, but may be significant with analgesic and anti-inflammatory doses of aspirin or other NSAIDs.[13]

In addition, acetylsalicylic acid and NSAIDs may cause the inhibition of platelet function and a subsequent increase in warfarin-associated bleeding risk. Augmentation of the anticoagulant effect of warfarin may occur with the use of paracetamol and salicylate doses of more than 1.5 g/day. On the other hand, cyclooxygenase inhibitors (rofecoxib and celecoxib) seem to have no significant effect on platelets or INR.[9]

INTERNATIONAL NORMALIZED RATIO MONITORING DURING DENTAL PROCEDURES

International normalized ratio must be measured prior to any dental procedure, ideally 24 hours before the scheduled procedure; however, in patients with stable INR, a measurement done within 72 hours of surgery may suffice. Evidence suggests that minor surgeries can be carried out safely within the therapeutic range (2.0–4.0) with the use of local hemostatic measures, to control bleeding. However, patients with an INR more than 4.0 are not advised to undergo any dental surgery without consulting the clinician responsible for managing their anticoagulation therapy.[6]

KEY POINTS

- Dental surgery on patients undergoing continuous anticoagulation is associated with the risk of bleeding from the procedure as well as the risk of thromboembolism due to the withdrawal of anticoagulation therapy
- Clinical evidence suggests against discontinuing or reducing anticoagulation therapy during minor dental surgeries, as the risk of thromboembolic events outweighs the risk of bleeding
- Invasive dental procedures may require stopping anticoagulation for 2–3 days before surgery and/or switching over to heparin, depending on the risk of thromboembolism
- Studies suggest that it may not be required to alter warfarin therapy in patients undergoing simple tooth extractions, provided the desired therapeutic INR range is maintained
- The use of NSAIDs as postoperative medication may affect the anticoagulant activity and increase the bleeding risk
- Minor dental surgery may be carried out safely within the therapeutic range of 2.0–4.0, provided local hemostatic measures are applied to control any bleeding event.

REFERENCES

1. Wahl M. Dental surgery in anticoagulated patients. Arch Intern Med. 1998;158(15):1610-6.
2. Martinez M, Tsakiris D. Management of antithrombotic agents in oral surgery. Dent J. 2015;3(4):93-101.
3. Mingarro-de-Leon A, Chaveli-Lopez B, Gavalda-Esteve C. Dental management of patients receiving anticoagulant and/or antiplatelet treatment. J Clin Exp Dent. 2014:e155-61.
4. Perry D, Noakes T, Helliwell P. Guidelines for the management of patients on oral anticoagulants requiring dental surgery. BDJ. 2007;203(7):389-93.
5. Bajkin B, Popovic S, Selakovic S. Randomized, prospective trial comparing bridging therapy using low-molecular-weight heparin with maintenance of oral anticoagulation during extraction of teeth. J. Oral Maxillofac Surg. 2009;67(5):990-5.
6. Pototski M, Amenábar J. Dental management of patients receiving anticoagulation or antiplatelet treatment. J Oral Sci. 2007;49(4):253-8.
7. Campbell J, Alvarado F, Murray R. Anticoagulation and minor oral surgery: Should the anticoagulation regimen be altered? J Oral Maxillofac Surg. 2000;58(2):131-5.

8. Sacco R, Sacco M, Carpenedo M, Mannucci PM. Oral surgery in patients on oral anticoagulant therapy: a randomized comparison of different intensity targets. Oral Surg Oral Med Oral Pathol Oral Radiol Endod. 2007;104(1):e18-21.
9. Evans IL, Sayers MS, Gibbons AJ, Price G, Snooks H, Sugar AW. Can warfarin be continued during dental extraction? Results of a randomized controlled trial. Br J Oral Maxillofac Surg. 2002;40(3):248-52.
10. Gacina P, Carzavec D, Stancic V, Pejsa V. Dental procedures in patients receiving oral anticoagulant therapy. Acta Clin Croat. 2006;45:101-4.
11. Abdullah WA, Khalil H. Dental extraction in patients on warfarin treatment. Clin Cosmet Investig Dent. 2014;6:65-9.
12. Devani P, Lavery KM, Howell CJ. Dental extractions in patients on warfarin: Is alteration of anticoagulant regime necessary? Br J Oral Maxillofac Surg. 1998;36(2):107-11.
13. Kharma MY, Sakka S, Aus G, Tarakji B, Nassani MZ. Anticoagulants and dental surgery: a review. Int J Dent Clin. 2015;7(2):28-31.

17

Bleeding Complications with Vitamin K Antagonists

Sridhar Kasturi

INTRODUCTION

Oral anticoagulant (OAC) therapy with vitamin K antagonists (VAKs) has been the mainstay of the treatment and prevention of thromboembolic complications in clinical conditions such as venous thromboembolism, atrial fibrillation, prosthetic valves, and ischemic stroke; however, the prophylactic efficacy of VKAs comes at the price of an increased risk of bleeding complications.[1] This chapter focuses on various factors contributing to increased bleeding risk associated with VKA therapy, the management and reversal of anticoagulation therapy, as well as the long-term evaluation of bleeding risk.

BLEEDING RISK WITH ORAL ANTICOAGULANTS

Bleeding associated with VKAs is one of the most important complications of OAC therapy that may influence the prognosis of treated patients, resulting in the potential discontinuation of therapy, morbidity, or even mortality.[1]

These bleeding events may include minor bleeds, such as short-lived episodes of epistaxis, or major life-threatening bleeds, such as intracranial bleeds.[2]

The maintenance of OAC therapy within a narrow therapeutic range is essential for increased protection against thromboembolic complications and a concurrent decrease in risk of bleeding events. An optimal international normalized ratio (INR) range of 2.0–3.0 has been suggested for most clinical conditions at increased risk of thromboembolic events; however, bleeding may manifest even with properly prescribed OAC. Although the interruption and/or withdrawal of anticoagulation therapy, along with the administration of coagulation factors, may be essential in the management of bleeding events, it is important to stratify patients, based on individual risk of bleeding, before initiating OAC.[1]

Factors that Increase Bleeding Risk with Vitamin K Antagonists

Several factors may contribute to an increased risk of bleeding during VKA therapy. These include individual patient characteristics and use of concomitant medications, as well as treatment factors such as the timing, intensity, and quality of OAC therapy (Box 1).[1]

Box 1: Factors associated with increased bleeding risk[1]

- Age >65–70 years
- Female gender
- *CYP2C9* and/or *VKORCI* gene polymorphism
- Higher intensity if anticoagulation (i.e., INR >4.5)
- Labile INR (i.e., TTR <60%)
- Early 90 days of anticoagulation
- Comorbidities (i.e., hypertension, malignancy, liver and/or renal and/or cardiac failure)
- Commedications (i.e., antiplatelet agents, nonsteroidal anti-inflammatory drugs)

INR, international normalized ratio; TTR, time within the therapeutic range.

Age

Evidence supports the link between old age and the increased risk of bleeding. A fivefold increased risk of major and fatal bleeding has been associated with the elderly compared to younger patients (3.2% and 0.64% per year vs 0.6% and 0.12% per year, respectively).[3] Various factors may lead to increased bleeding risks among the elderly, such as:[1]

- Reduced metabolic clearance, leading to reduced dose of anticoagulants required for effective anticoagulation
- Higher incidence of pathological changes in the cerebral vessels (increases the risk of intracranial hemorrhage)
- Increased prevalence of diverticulosis, ischemic colitis, angiodysplasias, and malignancy (which predispose to gastrointestinal bleeding)
- Higher prevalence of comorbid conditions and use of interacting drugs
- Higher rate of noncompliance

Comorbid Conditions[1]

Several comorbid conditions can potentially increase the risk of bleeding; these include:

- Previous episodes of bleeding
- Congestive heart failure
- Hepatic or renal failure
- Diabetes
- History of hypertension
- Malignancy, leading to INR fluctuations.

Comedication

Several drugs may have the ability to potentiate the anticoagulant activity of VKAs; the mechanisms by which they may do so include:[2]

- Decreasing VKA clearance
- Reducing the synthesis of vitamin K-dependent coagulation factors, and
- Increasing the clearance of vitamin K-dependent coagulation factors.

The major drug classes involved in increased bleeding include antibiotics, antifungals, antiplatelet agents, and nonsteroidal anti-inflammatory drugs (NSAIDs).[2]

The frequent coexistence of conditions such as venous thromboembolism or atrial fibrillation alongside coronary artery disease among the elderly, may often require the prescription of both VKAs and antiplatelet agents; this may result in an increased bleeding risk.[1] The concomitant administration of VKAs and aspirin has been reported to be associated with a relative risk of major bleeding of 2.5 [95% confidence interval (CI): 1.7–3.7].[4]

Genetics

Differential VKA sensitivity has been associated with mutations in *VKORC1*, and delayed stabilization of VKA therapy has been associated with *CYP2C9* polymorphisms. Patients with *CYP2C9* variants display unstable response to VKA, delayed achievement of dosage stability, supratherapeutic INR range during the initial treatment phase, and a higher risk of having an INR value of more than 5.0 compared to noncarriers, leading to an increased bleeding risk.[1]

Intensity and Quality of Anticoagulant Treatment

The therapeutic INR target is one of the major determinants of anticoagulant-related bleeding. An exponential increase in the rate of bleeding risk has been observed with INR values more than 4.5, while INR values between 2.0 and 3.0 have been associated with the lowest risk. A one unit increase in INR above 2.5 has been associated with a twofold increased risk of mortality.[1]

The time within the therapeutic range (TTR) depicting the quality of anticoagulation may also influence the risk of bleeding complications especially during the first 90 days of therapy initiation.[1] Significantly, higher rates of bleeding and mortality have been noted in patients with TTR less than 60% (3.85 and 4.20%, respectively) compared to those with TTR more than 75% (1.58 and 1.69%, respectively).[5]

Reversing the Anticoagulant Effect[6]

Various strategies may be used to reverse the anticoagulant effect of VKAs; these strategies include the administration of oral and intravenous phytonadione, fresh frozen plasma, and clotting factor concentrates. Fresh frozen plasma is derived from human blood and consists of all the vitamin K-dependent clotting factors present in the plasma.

The concentrated clotting factor reversal agents include:

- Three- and four-factor prothrombin complex concentrate (PCC) products
- Recombinant factor VII
- Activated PCC (aPCC).

These reversal agents differ in their clotting factor content. Table 1 lists the reversal agents and the respective clotting factors replaced by them.

Some PCC4 and aPCC agents may also contain natural regulatory anticoagulant protein C and/or protein S. As there is a potential risk of thrombosis associated with some of these clotting factor concentrates, weighing the risks against the benefits is, therefore, essential prior to using these products for the reversal of anticoagulation.

Table 1: Concentrated clotting factor agents and corresponding factors replaced during reversal of anticoagulation[11]

Reversal agent	Clotting factors replaced
PCC3	II, IX, and X (inactivated)
PCC4	II, VII, IX, and X (inactivated)
rFVIIa	VII (activated)
aPCC	II, IX, X (inactivated), and VII (activated)

rFVIIa, recombinant factor VII; aPCC, activated PCC, prothrombin complex concentrate.

MANAGEMENT OF BLEEDING[7]

The management of VKA-associated major and nonmajor bleeding complications involves the immediate discontinuation of VKA administration; however, the possible risks of thrombosis must be taken into consideration during the rapid reversal of coagulopathy. Flowchart 1 summarizes various strategies for the management of clinically relevant major and nonmajor bleeding situations.

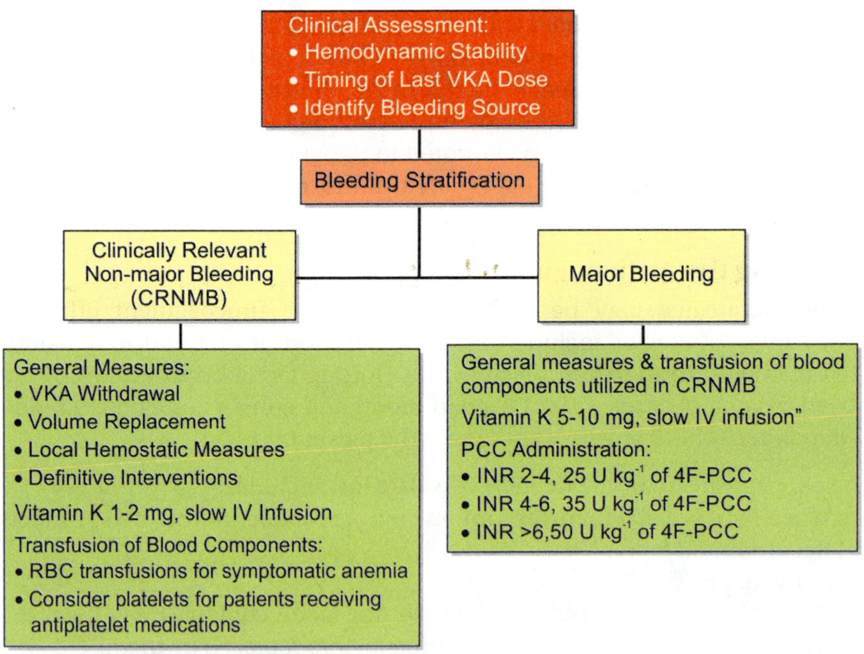

VKA, vitamin K antagonists; IV, intravenous; RBC, red blood cell; PCC, prothrombin complex concentrate; INR, international normalized ratio.

Flowchart 1: Management algorithm for vitamin K antagonists-associated bleeding[7]

*Lower dose vitamin K (1–2 mg) is considered for clinical conditions requiring early re-initiation of VKA therapy.

THE AMERICAN COLLEGE OF CHEST PHYSICIANS RECOMMENDS[8]

Rapid reversal of anticoagulation with four-factor prothrombin complex concentrate (PCC) with an additional administration of vitamin K (5–10 mg) through slow intravenous injection.

THE BRITISH COMMITTEE FOR STANDARDS IN HAEMATOLOGY GUIDELINES RECOMMENDS[9]

- Administration of 5 mg intravenous vitamin K and 25–50 U/kg four-factor PCC for emergency reversal of effect of acenocoumarol
- An oral vitamin K dose of 1–5 mg for correction of anticoagulation or for less severe bleeding.

LONG-TERM EVALUATION OF BLEEDING RISK

The incidence rates of bleeding during long-term VKA therapy are expected to be around 10–17% per annum for all events, with major bleeding events at around 2–5% per year and fatal bleeding events at around 0.5–1% per year. Intracranial hemorrhage, considered the most feared complication of bleeding, due to its association with high morbidity and mortality, has an incidence rate of 0.2–0.4% per year.[1]

A Spanish study documented 10-year experience with the use of acenocoumarol in ambulatory patients, with respect to hemorrhagic and thrombotic events. The most common indication for use of acenocoumarol in this cohort was atrial fibrillation. Overall, 73% of patients received acenocoumarol for atrial fibrillation. An analysis of 1,086 patients, with a median age of 74 years, receiving acenocoumarol showed that INR was in the therapeutic range (2.0–3.0) in 82.5% of patients. Overall, the bleeding rate (2.27/100 patients-year) and thrombotic event rate (0.2/100 patients-year) were low.[10]

KEY POINTS

- Bleeding is the most feared complication of oral anticoagulant therapy
- Several factors contribute to an increased risk of bleeding, such as age, comorbidities, concurrent medication, genetics, and the intensity and quality of anticoagulant treatment itself
- Clotting factor concentrates and fresh frozen plasma have been used for the reversal of the anticoagulation effect of vitamin K antagonists (VKAs) during bleeding complications
- The management of severe and life-threatening bleeding events through appropriate adjustments in international normalized ratio and the administration of appropriate clotting factor concentrates and oral vitamin K have been recommended for patients undergoing VKA therapy
- Long-term VKA treatment is associated with overall bleeding incidence rates of 10–17% per year
- A 10-year follow-up study with acenocoumarol treatment among the elderly showed a low incidence of bleeding complications.

REFERENCES

1. Rubboli A, Becattini C, Verheugt FW. Incidence, clinical impact and risk of bleeding during oral anticoagulation therapy. World J Cardiol. 2011;3(11):351-8.
2. Linkins LA. Bleeding risks associated with vitamin K antagonists. Blood Rev. 2013;27(3):111-8.
3. Keeling D. Duration of anticoagulation: decision making based on absolute risk. Blood Rev. 2006;20(3):173-8.
4. Rothberg MB, Celestin C, Fiore LD, Lawler E, Cook JR. Warfarin plus aspirin after myocardial infarction or the acute coronary syndrome: meta-analysis with estimates of risk and benefit. Ann Int Med. 2005;143(4):241-50.
5. White HD, Gruber M, Feyzi J, Kaatz S, Tse HF, Husted S, et al. Comparison of outcomes among patients randomized to warfarin therapy according to anticoagulant control. Arch Intern Med. 2007;167(3):239-45.
6. Nutescu EA, Dager WE, Kalus JS, Lewin JJ 3rd, Cipolle MD. Management of bleeding and reversal strategies for oral anticoagulants: clinical practice considerations. Am J Health Syst Pharm. 2013;70(21):1914-29.
7. Yates SG, Sarode R. New strategies for effective treatment of vitamin K antagonist-associated bleeding. J Thromb Haemost. 2015;13(Suppl 1):S180-6.
8. Holbrook A, Schulman S, Witt DM, Vandvik PO, Fish J, Kovacs MJ, et al. Evidence-based management of anticoagulant therapy: Antithrombotic Therapy and Prevention of Thrombosis, 9th ed. American College of Chest Physicians Evidence-Based Clinical Practice Guidelines. Chest. 2012;141(2 Suppl):e152S-84S.
9. Makris M, Van Veen JJ, Tait CR, Mumford AD, Laffan M; British Committee for Standards in Haematology. Guideline on the management of bleeding in patients on antithrombotic agents. Br J Haematol. 2012;160(1):35-46.
10. Trullas-Vila JC, Bisbe-Company J, Freitas-Ramírez A, Soler-Simon S, Bisbe-Company V, Roncero-Vidal JM, et al. Ten-year experience with acenocoumarol treatment in an ambulatory cohort of Spanish patients. J Thromb Thrombolysis. 2009;28(4):436-43.

18

Food and Drug Interactions

Sanjay Dhaded

INTRODUCTION

Vitamin K antagonists (VKAs), including warfarin, acenocoumarol, and phenprocoumon, are significantly effective and frequently administered for the prevention and treatment of thromboembolic diseases. However, several environmental and genetic factors, such as weight, sex, age, tobacco, and single nucleotide polymorphisms, influence the therapeutic response of the aforementioned oral anticoagulants.[1]

In most cases, patients receiving VKAs are also prescribed concomitant prescription drugs, over-the-counter medications, and dietary supplements. It is necessary to closely monitor the international normalized ratio (INR) while adding or withdrawing any medication, since polypharmacy can have an influence on the required dose of VKAs and enhance the risk of adverse events.[2]

In this chapter, we will discuss the food and drug interactions of VKAs.

FOOD INTERACTIONS WITH VITAMIN K ANTAGONISTS

Warfarin exhibits its anticoagulant effect by decreasing the amount of active vitamin K available for the activation of clotting factors II, VII, IX, and X.[3] It is believed that dietary vitamin K intake may counteract the anticoagulant effect of VKAs.[4] Warfarin response may vary with the dietary intake of vitamin K. Green leafy vegetables and certain vegetable oils contain a high amount of vitamin K. Foods containing a low amount of vitamin K may also become considerable source of the vitamin if their intake is increased. Several natural substances and foods that are reported to interact with warfarin are described in box 1.[5]

Box 1: Natural substances and foods reported to interact with warfarin[5]

- Potentiation of warfarin (increased international normalized ratio)
- Garlic
- Ginkgo
- Coenzyme Q
- Danshen
- Devil's clam
- Dong quai
- Ginseng
- Vitamin E
- Papaya

- Antagonism of warfarin (decresed international normalized ratio)
- Green tea
- Saint John's wort

DRUG INTERACTIONS WITH VITAMIN K ANTAGONISTS

Drug-drug interactions (DDIs) with VKAs can be categorized into 2 types: (i) pharmacokinetic and (ii) pharmacodynamic. In pharmacokinetic interactions, which occur in the majority of cases, the dose of VKAs must be adjusted. Pharmacodynamic interactions, e.g., the concurrent administration of antiplatelet drugs, may enhance the risk of bleeding without influencing the INR. The major classes of drug that have drug interactions with VKAs have been summarized in box 2.[2]

Box 2: Major drug interactions with vitamin K antagonists (VKAs): The 8 A's[2]

• Antibiotics	• Antiplatelet agents
• Antidepressants	• Acetaminophen
• Antifungals	• Anti-inflammatory drugs
• Amiodarone	• Alternative remedies

Drug-drug interactions are an additional factor that influences the variation of anticoagulation and the onset of serious adverse drug reactions.[1] Underlying mechanisms of DDIs include:[6]

- Disturbances of absorption
- Inhibition or induction of the metabolizing enzyme system (mainly Cytochrome P450 2C9)
- Reduced availability of vitamin K1, which is essential for the gamma-carboxylation of prothrombin complex factors.

Gschwind et al. conducted a study to determine the most clinically relevant DDIs that can affect the safety of acenocoumarol. The study used two different sources of information:

1. A 1-year retrospective analysis of acenocoumarol prescriptions and co-medications (n = 2,439 hospitalizations)
2. A retrospective study of clinical pharmacology consultations that involved acenocoumarol, from 1994 to 2007 (n = 407).

A criticality index for each drug was calculated by multiplying three parameters:

1. Mechanism of interaction
2. Involvement in a supratherapeutic INR (≥6)
3. Involvement in severe bleeding.[1]

The study noted 126 DDIs. The most frequent drug interactions with acenocoumarol that made it difficult to adjust the INR are depicted in table 1.[1]

A criticality index more than or equal to 20 was identified in 28 drugs (Table 2).[1] Based on a stratification of their mechanism of interaction, 14% of the drugs had a pharmacodynamic mechanism of interaction with acenocoumarol, while 75% of the drugs had a pharmacokinetic mechanism of interaction (in some cases, with an additional pharmacodynamic mechanism) (Table 3).[1]

Table 1: Drugs interacting with acenocoumarol in clinical pharmacology consultations for difficulty in adjusting the international normalized ratio[1]		
Supratherapeutic INR (n = 91) (%)	**Fluctuation of INR (n = 21) (%)**	**Subtherapeutic INR (n = 27) (%)**
• Amiodarone (11) • Acetaminophen (7) • Acetylsalicylic acid (5) • Clopidogrel (5) • Esomeprazole (4) • Simvasrarin (4) • Amoxicillin (3) • Clavulanic acid (2) • Ceftriaxione (2) • Fluconazole (2) • Voriconazole (2) • Others (53)	• Fluconazole (14) • Amiodarone (10) • Others (76)	• Carbamazepine (15) • Phenytion (7) • Rifampicin (7) • Others (71)
n = number of observations; INR, international normalized ratio.		

Table 2: Drugs with a criticality index of ≥20 International non-proprietary name[11]	
Criticality index	**International nonproprietary name**
640	Amiodarone
600	Acetylsalicylic acids
400	Esomeprazole
240	Clopidogrel
80	Paracetamol, Fluvastatin, Celecoxib
64	Fluvaxamine, Leflunomide
60	Ciprofloxacin
40	Escitalopram, Diclofenac, Omeprazole
30	Metronidazole
24	Clarithromycin, Simvastatin, Econazole
20	Prednisone, Fluconazole, Valproic acid, Ibuprofen, Lysine acetylsalicylate, Imatinib, Miconazole, Pantoprazole, Voriconazloe, Etodolac, Ketorolac

The author reported 28 specific drugs that are at high risk for interacting with acenocoumarol. Moreover, most of them interacted with acenocoumarol through the pharmacokinetic mechanism.[1]

> Most of the drug-drug interactions with vitamin K antagonists are through the pharmacokinetic mechanism.[1]

Sometimes, more than one mechanism is involved in DDIs. Importantly, any therapy can carry the risk of interaction, but every interaction is not

Table 3: Mechanism of interaction for the 28 drugs that exert a high risk of interaction with acenocoumarol (criticality index ≥20)[1]

PK mechanism	PD mechanism	PK and PD mechanism	Unknown mecahnism
• Amiodarone • Esomeprazole • Fluvastatin • Ciprofloxacin • Omeprazole • Metronidazole • Simavastatin • Econazole • Fluconazole • Valproate • Imatinib • Leflunomide • Micronazole • Pantoprazole • Voriconazole	• Etodolac • Ketorolac • Acetylsalicylic acid • Lysine acetylsalicylate	• Celecoxib • Fluvoxamine • Ibuprofen • Clopidogrel • Escitalopram • Diclofenac	• Clarithromycin • Prednisone • Paracetamol

PK, pharmacokinetic; PD, pharmacodynamics.

vital. Therefore, in patients receiving acenocoumarol, careful monitoring and frequent coagulation tests (twice weekly) should be considered while prescribing a new drug or while stopping a concomitantly administered drug.[5]

In patients receiving vitamin K antagonists, international normalized ratio should be closely monitored while withdrawing or adding a new drug to their regimen.[2]

KEY POINTS

- Certain foods and drugs can impact the pharmacokinetics and anticoagulant action of vitamin K antagonists (VKAs)
- Several drugs, including amiodarone, acetylsalicylic acid, esomeprazole, and clopidogrel, have been identified to have the highest risk of interaction with acenocoumarol
- Herbal preparations containing garlic, ginkgo, ginseng, vitamin E, papaya, and green tea have been reported to interact with VKAs
- Monitoring international normalized ratio, along with frequent coagulation tests, is required while starting a new drug or stopping a concomitantly administered drug in patients receiving VKAs.

REFERENCES

1. Gschwind L, Rollason V, Lovis C, Boehlen F, Bonnabry P, Dayer P, et al. Identification and weighting of the most critical "real-life" drug-drug interactions with acenocoumarol in a tertiary care hospital. Eur J Clin Pharmacol. 2013;69(3):617-27.

2. De Caterina R, Husted S, Wallentin L, Andreotti F, Arnesen H, Bachmann F, et al. Vitamin K antagonists in heart disease: current status and perspectives (Section III). Position paper of the ESC Working Group on Thrombosis—Task Force on Anticoagulants in Heart Disease. Thromb Haemost. 2013;110(6):1087-107.
3. Holbrook AM, Pereira JA, Labiris R, McDonald H, Douketis JD, Crowther M, et al. Systematic overview of warfarin and its drug and food interactions. Arch Intern Med. 2005;165(10):1095-106.
4. Violi F, Lip GY, Pignatelli P, Pastori D. Interaction between dietary vitamin K intake and anticoagulation by vitamin K antagonists: Is it really true?: A systematic review. Medicine (Baltimore). 2016;95(10):e2895.
5. Greenblatt DJ, von Moltke LL. Interaction of warfarin with drugs, natural substances, and foods. J Clin Pharmacol. 2005;45(2):127-32.
6. Trailokya A. Acenocoumarol in thromboembolic disorders. Cardiovasc Pharm Open Access. 2015;4(4):1-5.

19

Real-World Challenges with Anticoagulation

Rajiv Agarwal, Prashant Vaijyanath

INTRODUCTION

Vitamin K antagonists (VKAs) are the mainstay of the management of blood coagulation in patients with atrial fibrillation (AF), valvular heart diseases, venous thromboembolism, and valve replacements and in patients undergoing orthopedic surgery.[1] However, there exist some challenges in the optimal use of anticoagulant therapy. This chapter focuses on issues of concern in oral anticoagulant (OAC) therapy (particularly in India), patient- and physician-associated challenges to optimal anticoagulation, and the role of anticoagulant clinics in managing patients on anticoagulation.

CHALLENGES IN ANTICOAGULATION IN INDIAN SCENARIO[2]

Vitamin K antagonists are the most popular drug of choice for anticoagulant therapy in India. The availability of vast data proving the efficacy of VKAs over the years accounts for their widespread prescription. In addition, the high cost of drugs such as dabigatran makes VKAs the drug of choice in the Indian scenario. However, there are certain issues with the use of VKAs specific to the Indian population.

Diet

Indians vary in dietary habits compared to their Western counterparts. Inconsistency in the consumption of foods rich in vitamin K, such as green leafy vegetables, cabbage, and cauliflower, can lead to the underachievement of the target international normalized ratio (INR) in patients on VKA therapy and may result in INR fluctuations and related issues.

Over-the-counter Drug Usage

Indians frequently use over-the-counter medications such as nonsteroidal anti-inflammatory drugs (NSAIDs) or alternative herbal products, such as garlic and fenugreek, to cure certain ailments. These medications could accentuate the anticoagulation effect of VKAs and may result in bleeding complications. Certain antipyretics such as paracetamol and certain anti-tuberculosis drugs such as isoniazid can also lead to INR fluctuations and cause over or under coagulation.

Inadequate Monitoring

The lack of laboratories with standardized equipment to measure prothrombin time (PT)/INR in many Indian hospitals leads to the substandard monitoring of anticoagulation. Research regarding anticoagulation in the Indian setting suggests:

- Inferior outpatient anticoagulant control with poor pre-therapeutic assessment
- Unacceptably high number of subtherapeutic PT/INR values
- High rate of complications.

In addition, insufficient knowledge of target OAC among clinicians is also observed.

Genetic Factors

Recent pharmacogenetic findings validate the influence of genetic factors on the outcomes of OAC therapy. Large individual and ethnic variations in warfarin drug response have been reported. Three single nucleotide polymorphisms (SNPs), two in the *CYP2C9* gene and one in the *VKORC1* gene, have been found to significantly influence the effect of warfarin therapy on coagulation. The three SNPs identified aid in the determination of:

1. Warfarin dose required to produce a therapeutic INR (typically 2–13)
2. The risk of hemorrhage or of producing a supratherapeutic INR (>4)
3. The time required for the achievement of a stable therapeutic dose.

The importance of genetic variation, especially during the initial phase of OAC therapy, led the Food and Drug Administration, in 2010, to make specific recommendations for dosage range initiation in the carriers of *CyP2C9* and *vKorC1* gene variants as determined by genotyping testing. However, since no such testing is performed in India, it is hard to decide the accurate dosage of warfarin.

Ethnicity

As per a few studies done in China and Japan, Asians may require lower INR for protection against thromboembolism and may be subject to a higher bleeding risk at a lower INR compared to their Western counterparts. The lower body weight and body mass index of Indians may play a role in the lower dosage requirements. The influence of ethnicity with respect to warfarin dosage is lacking in anticoagulation consensus guidelines. In the Indian scenario, there exists insufficient evidence on VKA dosing risk and benefits.

Pregnancy

Since it is very common to detect pregnancy late in the first trimester in India, there is high chance of continuous warfarin use, due to lack of early briefing on the teratogenic effects of warfarin use during conception and pregnancy. Furthermore, implementation of guidelines suggesting low molecular weight heparin once daily prior conception is extremely difficult in India.

PHYSICIAN-RELATED CHALLENGES TO OPTIMAL COAGULATION[3]

Some of the practical issues faced by physicians in the day-to-day management of patients undergoing anticoagulant therapy include:

- Nonavailability of unifying and reliable source of practice guidelines and lack of information about advances in anticoagulant therapy
- Presence of clinically relevant differences in various stroke risk-stratifying schemes for patients with AF
- Lack of consensus among experts with respect to the most reliable tool for determining bleeding risk in patients with AF
- Uncertainty among physicians with respect to balancing the risk of thromboembolic event against risk of hemorrhage, leading to under-prescription of anticoagulant drugs.

Physicians often feel personally responsible for the therapy-associated bleeding risk, which negatively influences warfarin prescription. In general, physicians avoid prescribing warfarin due to the following reasons:[4]

- Perceived greater risk of bleeding
- Overestimation of the associated risks
- Underestimation of the stroke risk
- Clinical uncertainty about or inexperience with warfarin
- Perceived risk of noncompliance.

There is an apparent discrepancy between actual clinical practice and guideline recommendations, and anticoagulation is significantly underused in AF patients. To determine this, a questionnaire-based survey was conducted in Sweden wherein 728 physicians received a questionnaire on the Swedish guidelines for the management of AF. The results indicated that more than 94% of the physicians agreed with the recommendations regarding the long-term use of anticoagulants for stroke prevention in chronic AF patients at risk of thromboembolism. Despite this, of the 108 patients with chronic AF and at least one risk factor for stroke, and no contraindication for warfarin, only 40% received warfarin. Such noncompliance to guidelines may result in adverse outcomes and may affect patient quality of life and health care-related expenses.[5]

> There exists a discrepancy between guideline recommendations and actual clinical practice.[5]

Further, there is an underuse of OAC therapy in patients with AF with an elevated risk of stroke, in the real-world setting. A systematic review, which included 54 studies that linked stroke risk levels with the percentage of patients treated, indicated underuse of OACs in most high-risk patients, under treatment being defined as treatment in less than 70% of high-risk patients. Of 29 studies consisting of patients who experienced prior stroke/transient ischemic attack in need of OAC therapy as per published guidelines, 25 reported under treatment, with 21 of 29 reporting OAC treatment levels below 60% (range 19–81.3%). The study emphasized the need for improved therapies for the prevention of stroke in AF.[6]

> Underuse of anticoagulation therapy is prevalent in the real-world setting among patients with AF at elevated risk of stroke.[6]

PATIENT-RELATED CHALLENGES TO OPTIMAL COAGULATION

Several factors that are associated with non-adherence to warfarin therapy have been identified (Box 1). Although the risk of hemorrhage is higher among the elderly, it has been noted that younger patients are less adherent to warfarin therapy. Further, males and patients with a lesser risk of stroke also have lower warfarin adherence rates. Patients with a higher level of education tend to exhibit higher confidence in independent decision-making or decreased trust in physicians. Active employment also predisposes a patient to poor adherence to anticoagulation, on account of time restrictions. Similarly, poverty or the lack of resources is also a risk factor for poor adherence. Among medically ill patients, multiple factors associated with poor adherence have been identified; such factors include depressive symptoms, perceived lack of social support, impaired cognitive function, and poor health-associated quality of life.[7]

Patients demonstrate a wide variation in their preferences regarding warfarin therapy for stroke prevention. The various factors that may negatively influence patients on long-term warfarin therapy have been listed in Box 2.

Box 1: Factors contributing to noncompliance to warfarin therapy[7]

- Younger age
- Male sex
- Low overall stroke risk
- Poor cognitive function
- Poverty
- Homelessness
- Higher educational attainment
- Employment
- Reluctant receptivity of medical information

Box 2: Factors influencing quality of life of patients on long-term warfarin therapy[7]

- Inconvenience of taking the medication
- Inconvenience of frequent blood monitoring and clinic visits
- Preceived efficacy of the medication in preventing adverse outcomes (i.e., stroke)
- Anxiety related to potential and actual side effects of the medication
- Anxiety about potential drug-drug interactions
- Extent of shared decision making between the physician and patient when starting the medication
- Quality of information given to patients by physicians
- Impact of the medication on physical activities
- Dietary and alcohol restrictions

As per qualitative studies, the most commonly indicated difficulties among patients undergoing long-term warfarin therapy are restrictions on diet and consumption of alcohol, the burden of regular visits to the clinic, concerns about potential side effects, and drug-drug interactions.

There exists an apparent discrepancy in perceptions of risk, benefits, and impact on quality of life with long-term warfarin therapy among patients; this may significantly influence the pattern of medication compliance.[7]

A prospective cohort study was conducted to investigate the influence of patient adherence on anticoagulation control. The study included 136 participants observed over a mean period of 32 weeks and used electronic Medication Event Monitoring System (MEMS) medication bottle caps. The MEMS bottle caps recorded the exact time and date of pill bottle opening, thus monitoring warfarin usage. It was observed that:

- About 92% had at least 1 missed or extra bottle opening
- About 36% missed more than 20% of their bottle openings
- About 4% had more than 10% extra bottle openings.

In addition, the study findings also reported that each 10% increase in missed pill bottle openings was associated with a 14% increase in the odds of under anticoagulation ($p < 0.001$).

The study concluded that patients experience substantial difficulty in compliance with warfarin therapy; this, in turn, has a significant impact on anticoagulation control.[8]

ROLE OF ORAL ANTICOAGULANT CLINICS[9]

Anticoagulation clinics (ACs) provide specialized services for the management of anticoagulation. They may be a part of thrombosis center multifunctional services, with field experts providing expertise in the diagnosis and prophylaxis of thromboembolic diseases; or they may be an independent service provider. At present, ACs essentially manage patients on VKAs. Currently, four different management models are considered for patients on VKAs; these include:

1. Routine medical care
2. Anticoagulation clinics
3. Patient self-testing
4. Patient self-management.

Of the above four management strategies, ACs represent the best management model as indicated in table 1.

Table 1: Comparison of principal features of the four management models[9]

	RMC	AC	PSM	PST
Clinical quality	+	++++	++++	++++
TTR	+	+++	+++	++++
Accessibility	++++	++	+	++
Costs	+	++	+++	++++

RMC, routine medical care; AC, anticoagulation clinic; PSM, patient self-management; PST, patient self-testing; TTR, time in therapeutic range.

Anticoagulation clinics are involved in:

- Determining the correct indication for initiation of anticoagulation therapy
- Determining the appropriate laboratory testing needed for pharmacological monitoring
- Prescribing the correct anticoagulant treatment regimen, based on the test results
- Deciding appropriate time intervals for regular anticoagulation controls
- Assessing potential pharmacological interactions
- Assisting patients undergoing surgical interventions
- Conducting educational programs for patients and health care providers.

Advantages of ACs include:

- Specialized services with expertise in anticoagulant treatment and knowledge of coagulation mechanisms that can support patients even in critical conditions
- Provision of specific therapeutic intervention in case of emergencies, due to knowledge of complication etiopathogenesis
- Complete recording of essential clinical and laboratory data and easy accessibility to clinical surveillance and pharmacovigilance assessment.

KEY POINTS

- Vitamin K antagonists are the most popular drug of choice for anticoagulation in India
- Issues peculiar to the Indian scenario, such as diet, over-the-counter medication use, ethnicity, and genetic factors, may affect optimal anticoagulation
- Several physician-related factors influence optimal anticoagulation, including underprescription of anticoagulant medication
- Several factors contribute to noncompliance with warfarin therapy among patients, including patients' perception of the impact of long-term warfarin therapy on quality of life
- Anticoagulation clinics provide the best management model for the optimal treatment of patients on VKA therapy.

REFERENCES

1. Current Indian scenario on the use of oral anticoagulants. J Assoc Physicians India. 2014;62:28-9.
2. Gopalakrishnan S, Narayanan S. Oral anticoagulants: current Indian scenario. Medicine Update. J Assoc Physicians India. 2013:410-3.
3. Sen S, Dahlberg K. Physician's fear of anticoagulant therapy in nonvalvular atrial fibrillation. Am J Med Sci. 2014;348:513-21.
4. Lane DA, Lip GY. Barriers to anticoagulation in patients with atrial fibrillation: changing physician-related factors. Stroke. 2008;39:7-9.
5. Frykman V, Beerman B, Ryden L, et al. Medical Products Agency; Swedish Society of Cardiology. Management of atrial fibrillation: discrepancy between guideline recommendations and actual practice exposes patients to risk of complications. Eur Heart J. 2001;22:1954-9.

6. Ogilvie IM, Newton N, Welner SA, et al. Underuse of oral anticoagulants in atrial fibrillation: a systematic review. Am J Med. 2010;123:638-645.
7. Kneeland PP, Fang MC. Current issues in patient adherence and persistence: focus on anticoagulants for the treatment and prevention of thromboembolism. Patient Prefer Adherence. 2010;4:51-60.
8. Kimmel SE, Chen Z, Price M, et al. The influence of patient adherence on anticoagulation control with warfarin: results from the International Normalized Ratio Adherence and Genetics (IN-RANGE) Study. Arch Intern Med. 2007;167:229-35.
9. Testa S, Paoletti O, Zimmermann A, Bassi L, Zambelli S, Cancellieri E. The role of anticoagulation clinics in the era of new oral anticoagulants. Thrombosis. 2012;2012: 835356.

20

Role of Patient Education and Counseling during Anticoagulation Therapy

Ummer K, Bhupesh Shah

INTRODUCTION

Thromboembolic disorders are a significant cause of mortality worldwide. Anticoagulant therapy plays a crucial role in the management and prophylaxis of thromboembolic disorders. There exists a well-established association between patient education and superior anticoagulation control.[1] This chapter focuses on the role of patient education, counseling, self-management, and self-monitoring [through the use of at-home international normalized ratio (INR) monitoring devices] in the optimal management of anticoagulation.

ROLE OF PATIENT EDUCATION IN ANTICOAGULATION THERAPY

Evidence supports the association between patient knowledge and improved anticoagulation control. Frequent, well-defined patient educational programs for the management of anticoagulation lead to increased adherence to therapy and improved compliance. Good compliance in turns helps build patient confidence in therapy and minimizes therapy-associated complications. Good patient education provides necessary information in an easily understandable format and involves the patients as well as primary caregivers and family members.[1]

Patient education programs aim to influence patient attitudes toward therapy by improving knowledge, behavior, and practices leading to better health outcomes. The various techniques used to deliver patient education range from simple educational booklets to videos imparting additional information.[2]

The following key topics need to be addressed in any patient booklet:[1]

- What vitamin K anticoagulants (VKAs) are and why patients need them
- How VKAs work
- The importance of monitoring prothrombin time (PT)/INR
- Factors that can modify PT/INR
- Side effects of therapy
- Common medications and foods that can interact with the given anticoagulant and alter PT/INR
- Basic things to consider while on anticoagulation therapy
- Suggested course of action on experiencing complications such as bleeding
- Emergency contact information

In addition, on initiation of therapy, it is the physician's responsibility to discuss the implications of anticoagulant therapy, including risks and benefits, with the patient and their family members. Also, adequate time needs to be allotted to address any therapy-associated concerns raised by the patients or relatives. Relevant and comprehensive information related to the anticoagulant regimen needs to be provided beforehand.[1]

ACHIEVING OPTIMAL INTERNATIONAL NORMALIZED RATIO VIA PATIENT EDUCATION

Several factors might influence INR control, such as drug-drug interactions and variations in dietary vitamin K intake. Education interventions aim at encouraging behavioral change among patients by imparting adequate knowledge about the treatment and lifestyle factors involved in the therapy. This in turn helps patients maintain a therapeutic INR range.[2]

> Poor patient knowledge may result in poor INR due to intentional or unintentional nonadherence to anticoagulant therapy.[2]

Studies related to patient adherence suggest that poor INR may be a result of intentional nonadherence (when patients resist treatment due to personal beliefs and/or motivations) or unintentional nonadherence (when patients' skill or ability impacts medication adherence). Poor knowledge among patients with respect to their condition and/or their specific anticoagulant treatment regimen may influence their ability to manage treatment (unintentional) and their preconceived notions regarding treatment necessity (intentional).[2]

There is evidence suggesting a significant relationship between patient knowledge and time in therapeutic range (TTR), with greater TTR observed in more knowledgeable patients.[3] Therefore, educating patients on factors affecting their TTR and methods to manage their anticoagulant therapy may result in increased adherence to the therapeutic regimen. Adherence, in turn, has important clinical benefits, such as a reduction in adverse events like strokes and hemorrhage.[2]

PATIENT COUNSELING TO IMPROVE COMPLIANCE[4]

Managing patients on anticoagulant therapy such as warfarin is a challenging task for healthcare professionals. Suboptimal treatment has been reported in many studies. Continuous counseling and increasing patient awareness of various aspects of anticoagulant therapy will result in improved outcomes. For patients on chronic oral anticoagulation therapy, additional consultation through home visits or via phone calls may reduce hospital readmissions and result in improved compliance. In addition, studies suggest a 7-week counseling period in the majority of patients being discharged on oral anticoagulation therapy.

A comparative study consisting of 240 patients recently placed on warfarin therapy investigated the impact of continuous counseling on the outcomes of warfarin therapy and patient satisfaction. Accordingly, the patients were randomized to two groups: (i) the counseled group and (ii) the uncounseled group. The uncounseled group received the "usual medical care", whereas the counseled group was defined by the following criteria:

- Once-a-week telephonic consultation addressing a set of predefined questions
- Two home visits per month either by a nurse or a pharmacist
- Any additional consultation as per patient preference.

The results showed that the counseled group had significantly better INR control, fewer adverse events, and better patient satisfaction compared to the uncounseled group (Table 1 and Fig. 1).

Table 1: Comparison of outcomes between counseled group (Group A) and uncounseled group (Group B)[4]

Outcomes	Group A- Counseled group (n=120)	Group B- Uncounseled group (n=120)
Adverse effects		
Total number of adverse effects*	22	84
No. of patients experienceing adverse effects**	23	75
Events-thromboembolic/hemorrhagic		
Number of thromboembolic events	0	41
Number of hemorrhagic events	21	43
Hospital stay		
Number of hospital days used for warfarin adverse events	5	28
Median length of hospital stay in days*** (mean ± SD days)	3.2 (2.78 ± 0.85)	3.93 (5.32 ± 3.74)
Therapeutic range		
Admission INR outside therapeutic range	21	86
Subtherapeutic	11	33
Supratherapeutic	10	53

*p value = 0.0155, *p value = 0.0942, p value = 0.209.

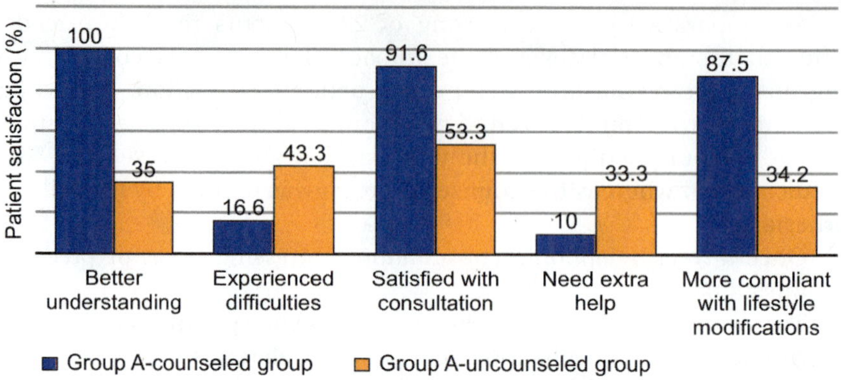

Fig. 1 Comparison of patient satisfaction between counseled group (Group A) and uncounseled group (Group B)

PATIENT SELF-MANAGEMENT AND SELF-MONITORING OF ANTICOAGULATION

Technological advances in anticoagulant management have led to improved anticoagulant management through point-of-care (POC) devices. The ease of use and portability of these instruments enable efficient self-assessment of INR. The inaccuracy involved in laboratory testing, due to the use of multiple reagents, has been minimized by the use of standardized POC instruments. Evidence supports the accuracy and precision of these devices, and they can be used to monitor both adults and children. Point-of-care devices are especially useful for patients under long-term anticoagulation therapy.[1] Patients can either self-manage their INR by adjusting their dosage as per a predetermined schedule, or they can self-monitor their INR and adjust the dosage according to that suggested by the clinician. The patients are usually trained in self-testing and provided instructions to prevent complications such as bleeding and thromboembolic events by their primary health care physician or nurse. Self-testing and self-management through portable monitors are established therapeutic practices in some countries such as Germany. These strategies of monitoring may be equal to or even better than standard monitoring by physicians, according to several published studies.[5]

Heneghan et al. investigated 14 randomized controlled trials (n = 3,049, mean age range: 42–75 years) that compared self-monitoring (self-test and/or self-manage) with management provided by anticoagulation clinics or the primary care physician of the patient (control group). The study findings showed that compared to the control group, the self-managed group had (Table 2):[6]

- Increased TTR
- Fewer complications of hemorrhage or thromboembolic events
- Lower mortality.

Table 2: Comparative analysis of selfmonitoring versus management by healthcare professionals in patients undergoing oral anticoagulant therapy[6]

Outcomes at 2–24 months	Thromboembolic event			Major bleeding				Death			
Self-monitoring category	Number of studies (n)	Weighted event rates		Self-monitoring category	Number of studies (n)	Weighted event rates		Self-monitoring category	Number of studies (n)	Weighted event rates	
		Self-moni-toring	Control			Self-moni-toring	Control			Self-moni-toring	Control
Self test	6 (1,341)	3.8%	6.5%	Self test	5 (1,191)	4.0%	7.0%	Self test	4 (1,028)	4.2%	5.1%
Self manage	8 (1,629)	0.8%	3.0%	Self manage	8 (1,629)	1.3%	1.4%	Self manage	6 (1,374)	1.1%	3.0%
Both	14 (2,970)	2.1%	4.6%	Both	13 (2,820)	2.5%	3.7%	Both	10 (2,402)	2.4%	3.9%

AT-HOME INTERNATIONAL NORMALIZED RATIO MONITORING DEVICES

Portable monitors for long-term anticoagulation monitoring, first introduced in the 1990s, allow patients to self-test their INR at home with a drop of whole blood. There are many POC devices available, such as ProTime® Microcoagulation System, INRatio® Monitor, Hemochron Junior Signature, and the Thrombolytic Assessment System near-patient test system; the most popular being the CoaguChek® monitor.[5] Several studies have established that POC testing and conventional laboratory-based techniques used by healthcare professionals are comparable in terms of their accuracy.[7-10]

Improved patient convenience, better compliance to treatment, more frequent monitoring, and fewer thromboembolic and bleeding complications are some of the potential advantages of self-testing and self-monitoring.[5]

IMPORTANCE OF PATIENT EDUCATION ON VITAMIN K FOOD INTAKE[11]

Patients on anticoagulation therapy must be counseled on the effect of dietary vitamin K intake on their treatment. A sudden increase in consumption of vitamin K-rich foods may decrease the effect of the anticoagulation treatment and may increase the risk of clotting, whereas a drastic and sudden decrease in dietary vitamin K intake may accentuate the anticoagulation treatment effect, thereby increasing the risk of bleeding. It is therefore advisable to keep the intake of vitamin K-containing foods consistent without any sudden increase or decrease in consumption. The recommended dietary allowance is 90 μg for women and 120 μg for men. Table 3 provides a list of foods containing moderate, high, and very high levels of vitamin K.

Table 3: Foods containing moderate, high, and very high amounts of Vitamin K[11]

Serving sizes are one cup unless otherwise noted—one cup is about the size of your fist		
Moderate (40–99 μg)	**High (100–400 μg)**	**Very high (401–1,200 μg)**
• Avocado (1 small to medium) • Asparagus (4 spears) • Broccoli, raw • Black eyed peas, cooked • Coleslaw • Edamame, cooked and frozen • Green leaf and romaine lettuces, raw • Okra, cooked	• Broccoli, cooked • Brussels sprouts, cooked • Cabbage, cooked • Butterhead and red leaf lettuces, raw • Plums/prunes dried, stewed • Radicchio, raw • Scallions, raw • Spinach, raw	• Beet greens, cooked • Collard greens, cooked • Kale, cooked • Mustard greens, cooked • Seaweed, dried (3.5 oz) • Spinach, cooked • Turnip greens, cooked • Dandelion greens, cooked